SURVIVAL OF
THE **FIRMEST**

UCLA Doctors Describe Ten Steps to
Better Erections, a Longer Life and
Reversing Erectile Dysfunction (ED)

David R. Meldrum, MD and
Joseph C. Gambone, DO, MPH

with

Marge A. Morris, M Ed, RD, CDE
and Claudia Meldrum

www.erectile-function.com

Foreword by Louis J. Ignarro, PhD
Nobel Prize Winner for Discovering
Nitric Oxide as the Key to Heart and
Erectile Health

Notice to Readers

Knowledge and best medical practices in the field of sexuality and male erectile dysfunction is constantly changing. Readers of this book and our website and other publications are advised to check the most current information provided by product manufacturers before undergoing any treatment. To the fullest extent provided by law, the authors and publishers of this book do not assume any liability for injury or damage to any individual or property arising out of or related to any use of the material contained in this book, our website or any recommended books or periodicals.

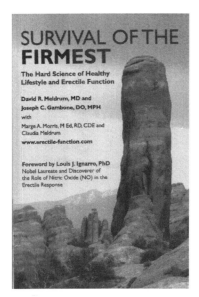

Previously published with cover to the left and recently revised and updated with current cover

The Meaning of
Survival of the **Firmest**

Early man was necessarily single-minded. He was frequently thinking only of how he could survive. When he wasn't sleeping he was hunting for food for himself and his family. And while he was hunting *he too* was being hunted by other animals trying to kill *him* for their own survival.

Regular physical activity was not a choice for early man—it was essential for his survival! Although he was not likely to live for more than twenty to thirty years at best, his body was firm, with good muscular strength throughout his short life. As long as he remained fit he could survive—an example of the *primary* principle of evolution theory—*SURVIVAL OF THE FITTEST.*

This fitness also allowed early man to survive long enough to produce offspring and pass his features on to them. But another kind of *fitness* or, more correctly, *FIRMNESS* must have been important for early man. Erectile health surely was an important factor because it allowed him to reproduce and pass this trait of *firmness* along with other genetic characteristics to the next generation. The rock formation pictured to the left has remained solid and firm over many thousands of years and serves as a symbol of a newer evolutionary principle—**SURVIVAL OF THE FIRMEST.**

This book provides factual information about natural and other safe medical methods to enhance and restore erectile health. Even more importantly, these same lifestyle changes and supplements will have a very favorable impact on survival and on overall health and vitality in general.

Foreword

Over the past two decades, research from our labora-tory and others has made the biochemistry and physiol-ogy of **Nitric Oxide (NO)** one of the most extensively researched and fundamentally important processes in the human body. Deficiencies of **NO** have been identi-fied in blood vessels ravaged by atherosclerosis, hyper-tension, obesity, high fat diets, and diabetes. Because exercise increases NO, the sedentary existence of most Americans also contributes greatly to poor vascular health. Although our work led to the discovery of Viagra, which has benefited countless millions of couples worldwide, Dr. Meldrum puts forth a potent argument in this book that we should not mask abnormal body chemistry and poor vascular function by simply treating the symptom (erectile dysfunction) with drugs. We now have the knowledge to correct the underlying problems leading to deficient **NO** production.

Just as I have emphasized in my nationally best-selling book *NO More Heart Disease*, the cardiovascular and gen-eral health benefits of enhanced **NO** synthesis by blood vessels has far-reaching benefits for each and every one of us. As Dr. Meldrum has pointed out, medicine should aim first to correct the underlying problems of disease. Simply trying to make up for the ravages of an unhealthy lifestyle by taking statins, using erectile stimulating drugs, or having cardiac bypass surgery will not address the underlying cause of the problem.

Dr. Meldrum's theory that the complex and redundant system of **NO** production evolved to assure firmness and erectile health for reproduction by early man is fascinating and compelling. It is an insight much like those that led to the invention of Velcro or Zip-lock bags—simple, yet one only has to examine its features to believe that it is true.

I have no doubt that this book will help millions of couples around the world by improving male sexual performance. It will also contribute significantly to the goal of my book *NO More Heart Disease.*

Louis J. Ignarro, PhD
Nobel Laureate, 1998

Ten Steps to Better Erections

In the following chapters wc will detail a fascinating process of personal discovery and a seven-year journey through the scientific literature that allowed us to assemble a ten-step process FOR ERECTILE HEALTH. Any man can improve his erectile function and his overall health and longevity by increasing nitric oxide (NO) production in the lining of his blood vessels naturally and safely, with the use of drugs only as needed. Here is a summary of what we found based on the hard science for improving erectile function.

Step 1

Get Moving
Nothing will make up for a lack of physical exercise. Sedentary men are up to ten times more likely to have problems with erectile function. Daily exercise stimulates vascular NO up to four-fold by a mechanical effect of the increased blood flow, by allowing insulin to stimulate NO more effectively, and by increasing one of the body's natural circulating antioxidants. Exercising pelvic floor muscles has been shown to help erections by keeping blood in the penis. Visit www.erectile-function.com for details.

Step 2

Increase Omega 3 Fatty Acids

Fish oil is the easiest and least expensive way to increase omega 3's, which stimulate NO 3-fold and stimulate other chemicals that relax blood vessels. Men with erectile problems can have serious existing or unrecognized vascular disease, and omega 3's prevent sudden cardiac death by stabilizing the heart's rhythm. We recommend 500 to 1,000 mg daily- not just the amount of fish oil- the amount of total omega 3's (EPA and DHA) listed on the label.

Step 3

Increase Antioxidants

NO is very unstable, lasting only a few seconds in tissues, and its production and stability require extensive antioxidant protection. Men with ED have decreased levels of cellular and circulating antioxidants. Strong antioxidants such as tea and chocolate increase NO and both have been shown to decrease the chance of a second heart attack. Berries and certain spices are also very potent sources. Pycnogenol is a commercial source of antioxidants similar to those in berries, and is well standardized. A dose of 50 to 120 mg per day would be a good substitute for or in addition to regular food sources. Antioxidants decrease blood pressure and are particularly important for men who smoke or have obesity or diabetes, all of which cause marked oxidative stress.

Step 4

Increase Folic Acid

Folic acid (folate) increases NO and prevents hypertension. Individuals are commonly deficient in this important vitamin. We suggest taking 400 micrograms daily unless dietary sources are clearly adequate. Green tea decreases folate in the body, making a 400 microgram supplement more important.

Step 5

Use It or Lose It—Penile Specific Exercise

Blood flow increases much more with erection than in the rest of the body with physical exercise. A study showed that ED was half as common in men who had more frequent erections. "Penile rehabilitation using a vacuum device or drugs is being increasingly used to preserve erectile function following prostate surgery. Use it or lose it!

Step 6

Quit Smoking and Avoid Smokers

Smoking causes marked oxidative stress and the production of toxic compounds that decrease NO production. Antioxidants appear to have the potential of reversing ED in smokers and preventing smoking-related vascular disease.

Step 7

Limit Alcohol

Excessive alcohol suppresses NO production by the lining of blood vessels and has been shown to cause structural changes in those same cells in the penis. Interestingly, excessive alcohol doesn't impair NO release from nerves supplying the penile blood vessels, explaining why strong sexual stimuli can still get it up in spite of a man being inebriated. Use of moderate alcohol, on the other hand, stimulates NO and is associated with a lower risk of ED. We don't advise starting to use alcohol, but keep it moderate (one or at the most two drinks). Red wine has the advantage of also containing stronger antioxidants, less sugar and fewer calories than beer.

Step 8

Lose Belly Fat

Abdominal fat causes insulin resistance, in part by releasing inflammatory factors that interfere with insulin's actions, one of which is to stimulate NO. Overweight individuals also ingest and burn more fuel, which releases free oxygen radicals and causes oxidative stress, further reducing NO. A low carbohydrate diet, exercise, and weight training to build more muscle will all decrease abdominal fat, lower blood pressure, increase NO, and improve erectile performance.

Step 9

Increase L-arginine and L-citrulline

The building blocks for NO are L-arginine in the diet and L-citrulline both in the diet and as a local source within cells. Doses of 5 grams of L-arginine or 2-3 grams of L-citrulline may improve erectile function and are more important for a vegetarian. Small doses of L-arginine such as 1 gram daily are commonly promoted but appear to be largely ineffective for improving erectile performance.

Step 10

Decrease Sugar and Fat

Sugar decreases NO production by blood vessels and the current American diet contains much too much sugar. Sugar is a moderately inexpensive way for the food industry to add flavor to foods and drinks. A high fat diet also suppresses NO, and both increase inflammatory factors involved in atherosclerosis and heart attacks. Many men ingest enough sugar and simple carbohydrates to be considered functionally diabetic and the typical high fat western diet regularly assaults a person's blood vessels. Importantly, antioxidants and exercise prevent many of the bad effects of fat and sugar on blood vessels.

What else?

If erectile function is not satisfactory after trying all these natural approaches, your physician should check a testosterone level and can give you a testosterone cream or patch if it is low. If you still need further help, Viagra or its long-acting cousins, Cialis or Levitra, will likely be effective but should be started at lower than usual doses. Once your blood vessels are producing more adequate amounts of NO, these drugs could cause a prolonged erection (over 3 hours can harm the penis) requiring a trip to the emergency room.

The prologue to the book and author's notes at the end of the book will provide a lot more detail and PubMed ID numbers you can easily cut and paste into Google so you can read the research summary. If you would like to read the individual papers, we'll tell you how to get them.

The rest is up to you. We have a self-evaluation available at www.erectile-function.com that will help to assure you are doing all you can to become the best lover you can be!

Below are references and their PubMed ID numbers for three reviews written by us together with Lou Ignarro,

PhD, who shared the Nobel Prize for the discovery of nitric oxide, and researchers from Naples, Italy who have published extensively on metabolism and erectile and vascular function.

David R. Meldrum, M.D., Joseph C. Gambone, D.O., M.P.H., Marge A. Morris, M. Ed., R.D., C.D.E., Louis J. Ignarro, Ph.D. A multifaceted approach to maximizing erectile function and vascular health. Fertility and Sterility 2010;94;214-220. [PMID:20522326]

David R. Meldrum, M.D., Joseph C. Gambone, D.O., M.P.H., Marge A. Morris, M. Ed., R.D., C.D.E., Donald A. Meldrum, M.D., Katherine Esposito, M.D., Ph.D., Louis J. Ignarro, Ph.D. The Link Between Erectile and Cardiovascular Health: The Canary in the Coal Mine. American Journal of Cardiology 2011, e-pub ahead of print 28 May 2011 [PMID:21624550]

David R. Meldrum, M.D., Joseph C. Gambone, D.O., M.P.H., Marge A. Morris, M. Ed., R.D., C.D.E., Katherine Esposito, M.D., Ph.D., Dario Giugliano, M.D., Ph.D., Louis J. Ignarro, Ph.D. Lifestyle and metabolic approaches to maximizing erectile function. International Journal of Impotence Research. 2011 (in press).

Table of Contents

Introduction

A Seven-Year Journey
Through The Medical Literature

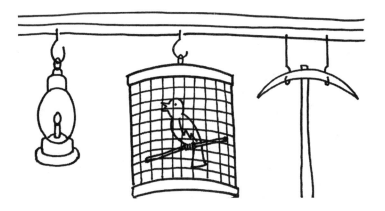

Up until as late as 1987, the canary was used as an early warning sign for British coal miners as a reliable and fairly inexpensive indicator of build-up of toxic gases in the mine in which they were working. The canary, with its rapid heart rate, was so sensitive to carbon monoxide and methane that it would stop singing and fall off its perch, allowing enough time for the miners to escape unharmed. This book describes a seven-year journey through the world's scientific literature culminating in a review article published in The American Journal of Cardiology in

August of 2011 highlighting poor erectile function as "the canary in the coal mine" for a man's heart and blood vessels. It has been increasingly realized that a man's erection is a very sensitive indicator of the health of the cardiovascular system. If a man's sexual performance markedly declines, particularly under age 60, it can sometimes be a critical warning sign of serious cardiovascular risk factors or unrecognized cardiac disease. In some cases, even sudden death could unexpectedly occur if the warning remains unheeded.

The world's medical literature is a fascinating conglomeration of over 5,500 journals of sufficient stature to be searchable through the National Library of Medicine. It is estimated that PubMed, NLM's electronic search portal, available to anyone on the planet with internet access, makes available scientific abstracts of close to a million research papers and reviews. A researcher with access through a university can retrieve the full version of most of these articles within seconds any time of the day or night. Each of those articles, besides giving the authors' findings, discusses most of what had been found on the subject up until that point and provides a reference list of relevant published papers. This allows a researcher to scour the world's literature to an extent that previously would have been simply impossible by searching through printed journals of even the best biomedical library.

Throughout this book we will give the PubMed ID numbers for the studies we quote, which can be pasted into Google's search field. Google will then take you to the pertinent summary of the article if you want to review the actual results. If the paper itself is desired, your local library may be able to provide it for you at a nominal charge. Lonesomedoc (1) is an electronic service set up by PubMed allowing access to full papers through a nearby medical library (2). For example, anyone can register through UCLA and request an electronic version of an article for $11 U.S.

What soon became apparent as my co-authors and I began this journey was that for this particular topic, the findings were buried among a very large number of journals. Often the importance of the findings was much greater than the recognition offered by those journals and sometimes greater than even the authors themselves seemed to have realized. Scattered throughout the world's journals were findings of major importance for the cardiovascular system, and by bringing all of those findings together, it was possible to assemble the cohesive story that will be described in this book. The final ninety-two references considered to be the most important for the review were drawn from fifty-seven different medical journals.

It also rapidly became apparent that lifestyle and nutritional factors have profound effects on both erectile and cardiovascular health and that the central mediator of those effects on blood vessel health is a fascinating gas called nitric oxide (NO). Hence the title of our review: "The Link Between Erectile and Cardiovascular Health: The Canary in the Coal Mine." That link, of course, is NO.

Who would ever have imagined that a gas would be identified as one of the body's most important signaling molecules and as having such profound effects on the vascular system? For many years it was recognized that a substance produced in the lining of all blood vessels (the endothelium) relaxes the smooth muscles around those vessels (called endothelium-derived relaxing factor, or EDRF) and keeps blood pressure in the usual normal range. If the blood vessels constrict, therefore not allowing enough blood flow to a tissue or organ, the effects understandably can be severe, resulting for example in a heart attack, a stroke, or kidney disease. For the penis, which relies on a very large increase in blood flow to provide the engorgement necessary for an erection, it's disastrous. A man can have a persistent inability to have an erection sufficient for satisfactory sexual performance (termed erectile dysfunction, or ED) or, more often, an age-related gradual decline in sexual performance impairing but not eliminating a man's sexual ability.

As a result of extensive research in laboratories all over the world, NO was finally conclusively identified as being the elusive EDRF. That discovery was of such fundamental importance that the 1998 Nobel Prize for Physiology and Medicine was awarded to Robert F. Furchgott, Louis J. Ignarro, and Ferid Murad. We were extremely fortunate to have Lou Ignarro, PhD, as the senior author for our review. Lou has described his journey toward that discovery in a fascinating national best-selling book called *NO More Heart Disease*, available through Amazon and any major book store. It's a great read for anyone interested in the key milestones in medical history.

One of Lou's many contributions to elucidating the role of NO in vascular health was by defining its role in the human erectile response. Using human penile tissue, he and his fellow investigators at UCLA showed conclusively that when the nerves supplying the penile tissue were stimulated, NO was released by those nerves to cause the increased blood flow necessary for erection (NO release from the penile nerves causes the "turned on" feeling a man gets when sexually aroused). They also showed that NO acted on the penile tissue through a cellular signaling system called cyclic GMP. People are more familiar with cyclic AMP as the mediator of the many effects of caffeine, and just as caffeine inhibits the breakdown of cyclic AMP, they were able to show that an inhibitor of the breakdown of cyclic GMP caused the effect of NO on the penis to be enhanced. Their work therefore led directly to the development of Viagra and other inhibitors of cyclic GMP degradation, Cialis and Levitra, which have helped many millions of men world-wide with ED. Their landmark article was published in the prestigious *New England Journal of Medicine* in 1992 (PMID: 1309211).

My own long journey began with an observation. If a researcher is very, very lucky and keeps his or her eyes, ears, and mind open, a simple observation can be the catalyst to begin a process of scientific inquiry. I had been researching nutrition because of my concern about the rapidly increasing weight in my infertility patients and the suspicion, now amply demonstrated, that obesity was contributing to their difficulty conceiving. I became particularly interested in the omega-3 fatty acids, which are obtained by eating fatty fish such as salmon, sardines or herring, or by taking fish oil supplements. They are essential, meaning they are not made by the body and must be obtained in the diet. Most people are deficient in these important nutrients.

One of the key references in our review was published following a detailed analysis of the health-promoting effects of omega-3s by the American Heart Association Nutrition Committee in 2002 (PMID: 12438303). The omega-3s have anti-arrhythmic effects on the heart muscle and had been observed to decrease sudden cardiac death, presumably due to their rhythm-stabilizing effect following a heart attack. They also have anti-inflammatory effects and inhibit platelet adhesion, which could also limit the severity of a heart attack. It is now recognized that inflammation is a key force causing rupture of atherosclerotic plaques in the arteries supplying the heart. Adhesion of platelets also contributes to narrowing of a coronary artery enough to cause a heart attack.

The omega-3s have also been shown to lower blood pressure (PMID: 2137901). The American Heart Association recommends taking a gram of omega-3s for any person with established coronary artery disease (CAD). I'd had my share of margarine, steaks, and fries when I was younger and figured my blood vessels could use the help that the omega-3s might provide.

I began taking a gram of omega-3s per day and started to observe a very pleasant side effect. I had been approaching age sixty, and just as with most men of that age, I had begun observing less sexual interest and ability. My wife and I have always been very sexually active and it was becoming a bit of a chore to keep up our customary schedule of activity. Within a few weeks of beginning the omega-3 supplement, and with no other apparent change in diet or my stress level or amount of sleep, I was feeling like I was twenty-five again! There was absolutely no question that I was experiencing marked increases in both sexual desire and performance. Having been aware of Lou's research, I suspected that NO might be involved and quickly found articles showing an increased production of NO in association with a higher consumption of omega-3s.

In an in vitro study (PMID: 9125207) one of the two principal omega-3s was added to human endothelial cells, and the level of NO production increased about three-fold! Further research revealed that folic acid (a vitamin) is an important additional ingredient in NO production, and that calcium and antioxidants (present in large amounts in fruits, vegetables, and some other foods) are also important for maintaining NO release. My diet has always included good amounts of all of these nutrients, and I also have maintained a low fat intake (fats decrease the NO production that normally occurs in the lining of blood vessels).

However, I was not currently taking additional folic acid as a supplement.

Folic acid, or folate, is also known to increase NO and improve heart and blood vessel health. In a study published in the *Journal of the American Medical Association* in 2009, folic acid was shown in women to decrease subsequent development of high blood pressure (PMID: 19622819). I decided to begin taking an 800 microgram supplement of folic acid. Whether it was adding the folic acid or just the cumulative effect of the omega-3s over time, I began to feel even younger than twenty-five, which was interesting but not particularly desirable. Since then I have reduced my total dose of omega-3s to between 500 and 1,000 mg including my already high seafood diet, and I have reduced my folic acid supplement to 400 micrograms per day, which keeps me feeling a manageable twenty-five years old. At the same time I must admit that I am performing in ways that are superior to anything in my experience throughout my life. Needless to say, as any man would be, I am very pleased with my response and with the benefits of having a better understanding of the biochemistry of NO. I have definitely not heard any complaints from my wife!

Thus began my long and arduous journey through the literature, gathering information about the various factors influencing NO production by blood vessels. I must admit that through most of that process of discovery I had a very strong prejudice that the Viagra-like drugs were simply treating the symptom (ED), while doing nothing to solve the underlying problem of decreased NO production by blood vessels. Besides producing an erection, NO has many positive effects on vascular health. It inhibits the ability of white blood cells and platelets to stick to the blood vessel lining (an initial step in formation of fatty plaques), opposes the growth of muscle surrounding the blood vessel, helps maintain normal tone of the muscle and therefore a normal blood pressure, and acts as an anti-inflammatory agent and reduces oxidative stress, two further factors involved in the formation of fatty plaques that constrict the passage of blood through the vessel and cause "hardening of the arteries."

It seemed to me at the time that use of drugs for ED was just one further example of a medical treatment for the symptom rather than the underlying disease, such as open heart surgery to fix cardiac blood vessels ravaged by an unhealthy lifestyle. As we will describe, that initial prejudice against the PDE-5 inhibitors (Viagra and its cousins inhibit the action of phosphodiesterase-5 that breaks down cyclic GMP) turned out to be unwarranted because of some startling new findings we'll discuss.

So what can every man do to optimize NO production in his blood vessels to improve both his erections and his overall health? After reviewing hundreds of articles, we were able to assemble a remarkable story of the profound influence of lifestyle and nutrition on vascular health, described in our journal review (3). At the beginning of this book we briefly listed ten steps to better erectile function and in notes at the end of the book we will describe in much greater detail what we consider to be these ten most important things you can do to maximize your erectile potency.

Back to where this all began—that keeping up my wife's and my usual schedule was becoming a chore? Well, that's a distant memory. Our love life is much better even compared to when we were first together, and it keeps on getting better. At first it was difficult to believe, but now that I fully understand the biochemistry of NO it all makes perfect sense. With erections, we're dealing with a system designed with multiple redundant pathways to be sure that this vital function will reliably occur, which gives us multiple interventions to improve NO production. Add in the ability to block the breakdown of cyclic GMP using drugs, and the likelihood of achieving excellent erectile function is within reach of most men experiencing difficulties. Unfortunately there will be instances where disease of the blood vessels or other problems such as treatments for prostate cancer will make an adequate response difficult or impossible, but even then there are approaches available that will be discussed in other chapters.

Back to the Canary

One thing that became very clear as we researched this subject was that a marked and consistent decrease of erectile function can be a critical warning sign of cardiac risk factors, possible underlying coronary artery disease, and risk of serious cardiac events even including sudden death. Now we don't want every man who has had occasional difficulty performing to rush out to see a cardiologist, but if the dysfunction is consistent and severe, men who are under age sixty (particularly under age fifty), and men with diabetes or hypertension should have a thorough evaluation by their physician. Also, better control of diabetes or hypertension is associated with improved erectile function. The longer these diseases continue to remain uncontrolled, the less chance that you will respond to any of the treatments we recommend, including the PDE-5 inhibitors. Also, the sooner that erectile function improves, the more likely the frequency of erections will also improve and help you to maintain your erectile health. For high blood pressure, there is good evidence that the short-acting angiotensin receptor blockers (ARBs) will actually improve erectile function. They appear to have an ancillary effect in reducing oxidative stress.

We've all heard how people corner a doctor at a cocktail party and start asking questions about their private health problems. Well, I've never experienced much of that, but purely by coincidence I recently met a fellow pilot about fifty years old (we'll call him Ted) who got around to asking me whether Viagra, Levitra, or Cialis was better for ED. Not having tried them, I couldn't give an opinion, but I did tell him about this book and shared my recipe for erectile health with him. At the time he had a girlfriend and was concerned that he "couldn't keep up with her" even with prescription medical assistance. We'll check in with Ted throughout the book to see how he's doing.

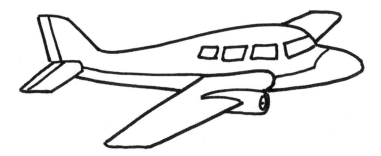

Chapter One

How an Erection Happens

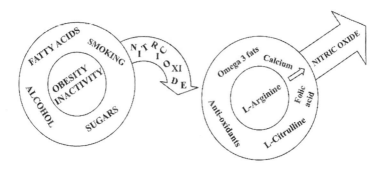

You have probably heard of the "fight or flight response"—our bodies' natural reaction to perceived danger. This reaction happens because our bodies are influenced by the sympathetic part of the nervous system that prepares the body to react to a threat by either staying to fight or by fleeing the area—fight or flight. A big part of this protective response involves the shifting of blood and oxygen from less important areas, such as the digestive and reproductive systems, during an emergency and directing them to the heart, muscles, and brain, providing the physical power and the wits to deal with danger. Another portion of our nervous system, called the parasympathetic part, does the opposite by shifting blood and oxygen to the less critical areas when the environment is free of danger and suitable for eating and reproducing.

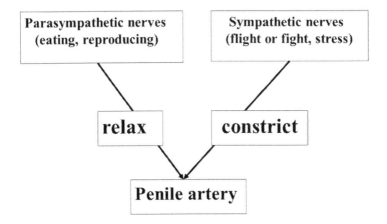

For the penis to fill with blood and become erect, the parasympathetic nerves responding to sexual stimuli that we see, feel, hear, smell, or even imagine cause the arteries in the penis to relax. Dr. Louis Ignarro, a UCLA researcher who won the Nobel Prize in Medicine in 1998 has clearly shown that a substance called nitric oxide (NO) is largely responsible for the relaxation of the penile arteries. We will use the abbreviation NO throughout the rest of the book. The body's production of NO thus results in increased blood flow into numerous tiny blood sacs in the penis called sinusoids. As a result, blood flow into the penis increases thirty to forty fold. The penis becomes engorged with blood and enlarges. This increased size then puts pressure on the penile veins. This pressure prevents outflow of blood from the penis and allows the erection to last. The firmness of the erection thus depends on the amount of blood entering the penis permitted by the relaxation of arteries and smooth muscle around the sinusoids. This healthy situation allows the penis to become engorged and erect.

The sympathetic nerves, on the other hand, cause the smooth muscle to constrict, significantly reducing blood flow. This lack of engorgement and erection is helpful when fighting or fleeing from danger but not so helpful when an erection is desired and safe to have. We can easily see how stress, by activating the sympathetic nerves, so readily prevents an adequate erection, or does not allow an erection to last long enough to satisfy both partners.

Basically there are two requirements for an erection to happen. First, sexual stimuli that we see, feel, smell, hear, or imagine must stimulate parasympathetic nerves to release NO and other substances such as prostaglandin E1. Together these substances relax penile smooth muscle and allow the penis to become engorged with blood. Second, there must be a fairly low level of sympathetic nerve stimulation (stress), which at higher levels would cause the smooth muscles to contract and prevent blood from filling the penis.

The various factors providing adequate sexual stimulation are complex and vary widely among individuals. In order to have healthy erections, any stressors that may activate the sympathetic nerves and cause constriction of penile smooth muscle should be kept at a minimum. This is why we need to be in the right mood, and why worries about the office or finances, for example, can spoil that mood and our sexual performance so easily. The role of stress has been widely recognized, and most men have probably observed that stress is a nonstarter when it comes to an adequate erection. Web MD has an excellent discussion of the role of stress in ED and how to limit its effects (www.webmd.com/content/article/57/66246.htm).

The effects of NO and stress are illustrated below.

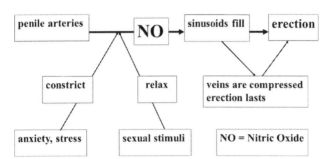

Nutrition plays a major role in allowing the right chemical conditions for enough NO to be released (see Chapter Six, "Good Nutrition Makes for Good Sex"). NO then stimulates production of the chemical that initiates smooth muscle relaxation, called cyclic guanosine monophosphate (cyclic GMP—see the diagram below). Prescription drugs such as Viagra, Levitra, and Cialis can only attempt to raise the levels of cyclic GMP by decreasing its breakdown. If there is very little NO and cyclic GMP being produced in the body, decreasing its breakdown will not work to raise the levels high enough to allow for an adequate erection.

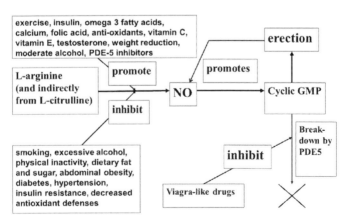

NO is produced from L-arginine, an amino acid formed by the breakdown of certain proteins. NO production is increased by antioxidants, folic acid, omega-3 fats, and calcium and decreased by high levels of fatty acids and sugar circulating in the blood. This commonly happens in individuals on a high-fat or high-sugar diet or with obesity and diabetes. NO then stimulates cyclic GMP, which causes penile smooth muscle relaxation, engorgement with blood, and erection. An enzyme, phosphodiesterase 5 (PDE 5), breaks down cyclic GMP. Viagra and other Viagra-like drugs raise the levels of cyclic GMP by inhibiting or decreasing its breakdown.

Prostaglandins also have some role in relaxing the smooth muscle in the penis. Injection of prostaglandin E1 (Caverject) into the penis is effective in about 60 percent of ED cases and allows for an erection in five to fifteen minutes. A suppository form (Muse) is also available. It is placed into the urethra and its effectiveness is similar to the injectable form (see Chapter Four, "When Nature Needs Help – Treatment Choices for ED").

The effectiveness of prostaglandin E1 suggests that low-dose ("baby") aspirin might be of benefit for ED. Low-dose aspirin tips the balance of various prostaglandins toward smooth muscle relaxation, a benefit for erectile health, and has been found to increase pelvic blood flow in infertile women. Low-dose aspirin is commonly used by men over the age of fifty or with cardiovascular disease to prevent heart attacks. It has not been studied for its effect on male potency, however. Although low-dose aspirin may be of only theoretical or limited benefit for ED, it certainly should not be harmful for erectile health.

"Something very interesting is happening here. Since taking these supplements, I've not only had better erections, but my desire has really increased. Things that haven't gotten me aroused for many years now do, and I find myself thinking about sex much more often, like when I was a young man. Someone should measure male hormone levels before and after these supplements. I bet they're higher." — Anonymous

If all this sounds a bit too complicated, just remember that sexual arousal causes blood vessel relaxation and an adequate erection, and the factor most responsible is NO. Antioxidants, folic acid, omega-3 fats, and calcium all help NO production, while high fatty acid and sugar levels decrease NO production. NO allows for erection through the effect of cyclic GMP. Prescription drugs like Viagra, Levitra, and Cialis increase cyclic GMP levels by decreasing its breakdown. Stress reduces blood flow into the penis by constricting the penile artery. Therefore good nutrition improves NO production and erectile health, and obesity and a high-fat and high-sugar diet decrease NO production and erectile health. Excess stress can undo it all. We'll show you how to keep NO production high to improve erectile health. Although decreasing stress will be primarily up to you, there are further suggestions that should be helpful on our website at www.Erectile-Function.com.

Ted had tried the omega-3s and the folic acid. He wasn't doing very well in increasing his activity, but at least he was not overweight. He was not yet taking much in the way of natural antioxidants, so I suggested taking 500 mg of vitamin C and 200 units of vitamin E daily. Out of the blue, I received an e-mail from pilot Ted:

I would like to thank you for sharing your recipe with me for erectile dysfunction. I have taken your prescription since the first week of February 2006. At first I was skeptical but decided to try. I have to admit that there are a few areas of your recipe that I need to work on. In spite of that, within three weeks I started to get erections in the middle of the night whereas before I would be lucky to get a half hard one. NO FUN! About the fifth week, when I would see a suggestive picture or movie I would start to get aroused. GOOD FEELING.

My thought is: with the results I am receiving by not following your recipe 100%, just think of how much better it would be if I made a valid effort to follow it as prescribed!

It's unfortunate that I haven't been able to test fly your recipe with a partner. I can only do ground runs. I will inform you if I get a test flight and how good the ride is.

My thanks again.
And a happier man,
"Ted"

References:

1) Rajfer J, Aronson WJ, Bush PA, Dorey FJ, Ignarro LJ: Nitric oxide as a mediator of relaxation of the corpus cavernosum in response to nonadrenergic, noncholinergic neurotransmission. New Engl J Med 1992;326:90-4.

Chapter Two

Extra Fat – It Can Ruin Your Health

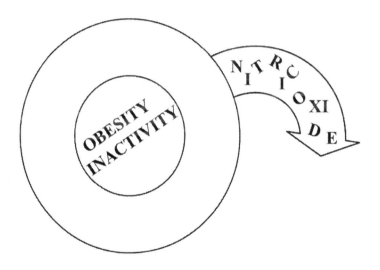

At first it might seem surprising that simply having extra fat can cause erectile dysfunction (ED). If being overweight or obese only meant that the body stores too much fat, one might suppose that the fatigue and depression often experienced by those who are overweight or obese are the only reasons for erectile problems. It turns out that the impact of significant excess body fat on erection is much greater. An obese person's metabolism is so completely out of whack that there are a number of other likely mechanisms.

Fat cells do much more than simply store extra fat. First they respond to increased calories by expanding their numbers to as many as one hundred billion cells. They produce inflammatory compounds such as tumor necrosis factor alpha (TNF-alpha) and interleukin-6 that promote inflammation in blood vessel walls, decreasing blood supply to tissues. Increased secretion of TNF-alpha and reduced secretion of adiponectin by fat tissue contribute to the body's reduced response to insulin (insulin stimulates the production of NO, the main mediator of the erectile response). Insulin resistance and sugary drinks and foods raise the blood sugar level, and these higher levels of sugar reduce the production of NO by the blood vessel lining. Diabetic men have a nearly three times greater incidence of ED. Fat cells are constantly breaking down fat to form free fatty acids, which in turn decrease the production of NO.

Fat cells also produce compounds such as angiotensinogen, which promotes constriction of blood vessels. This is exactly the opposite of the relaxation and increased blood flow needed for erection to occur and to last long enough for satisfactory intercourse. Excess fat cells are surrounded by a huge number of blood vessels, drawing much needed blood away from important activities like filling the penis with blood to cause an erection. A *large* waist truly is a *great waste*!

Overweight individuals eat more unhealthy food (see below), and the burning of that fuel releases more free oxygen radicals that interfere with NO production. Natural NO production is one of the most important chemical reactions for erectile health, and eating too much food poisons this process.

And finally, obese individuals are often inactive physically because of the fatigue they feel from carrying their extra weight. As a result of this decrease in physical activity, an obese man's circulation loses its ability to respond with increased blood flow. This high blood flow is essential both for the physical exertion required for him to have intercourse and for his penis to become engorged with blood and remain erect during intercourse. It is hardly surprising that obesity is associated with poor erectile health. In fact, it's amazing and actually very fortunate that all obese individuals do not have severe ED.

The really good news is that in a scientific study of 110 non-diabetic obese men, simply losing weight and increasing physical activity improved erectile health in one out of three of the men. A more aggressive approach to better nutrition and physical exercise would probably help many of the others. Diabetes presents a more difficult problem but there is help for diabetic men too.

So what should you do if you have ED? It turns out that the exact same habits that promote overall good health—eating a nutritious diet, losing weight if you are overweight, and having a physically active life style—will improve most of the negative factors that can interfere with a satisfying sex life. And if you can look forward to good sex on a regular basis, perhaps you will not miss the extra food you were eating!

Some Common Myths about Obesity

We've all heard it said over and over, "People are fat because they eat too much." Actually quite the opposite is usually the case. People for the most part eat too much *because they are fat*. If we consider that an obese person weighs at least one and one-half times as much as a normal person, s/he will require one and a half times as many calories just *to maintain that extra weight*. S/he has many more cells to feed and a much larger and heavier body to move around. Compared to the average requirement of 2,000 calories per day for a person of normal weight, an obese person is consuming at least an extra 1,000 calories (a total of at least 3,000 calories) *because of* their larger size.

Now that two-thirds of the U.S. population is overweight, typical portion sizes have increased to satisfy these much larger appetites. In the 1950s a bottle of Coke contained 6.5 ounces! Today a glass of cola is at least 12 ounces, and it is common for consumers to buy products containing as much as 32 ounces of soft drink. We recently saw a 42-ounce sugar-containing soda advertised for 69 cents in the window of a fast-food outlet! Typical restaurant meals are enough for two normal-sized people. Food plates are often larger to hold these bigger portions, and it is well known that when a dish is larger, a person tends to place more food on it.

All of these factors of daily living make it more diffi-cult for smaller people (especially women) to control their weight. This is true because the amount of food they need to eat to maintain their normal weight is so much less than the total calories in the food portions that are typically offered to them at meal time. This is particularly true in American restaurants. Bigger is better—but is it really? For people who are of normal weight, staying that way is becoming more and more difficult.

The increased calorie requirement of a heavy person makes it more difficult for him/her to lose weight. Not only does that person have to reduce his/her food intake by five hundred calories per day to lose fifty pounds in a year (a realistic weight loss goal of about a pound per week), but for each ten-pound weight loss, they will have to trim another eighty calories from their daily diet (eight calories for every pound lost) because there is less body tissue to feed and a lighter body to move around. In addi-tion to the five hundred fewer calories to **lose** the weight, that person has to trim another eighty calories per day as each ten pounds are lost so that they continue to lose at the same rate, and they will have to adjust to eating less food (in this example, a total of 50 lb. x 8, or 400 fewer calories per day) just to maintain their weight once the fifty pounds are gone.

Permanent weight loss is not easy! It is very important for people who want to lose weight and keep it off to eat foods that are lower in calories but also filling. This is necessary in order to satisfy their appetite in spite of the lower number of calories consumed. Otherwise people attempting to lose weight are likely to give up because they constantly feel hungry.

And so in a very real sense people don't *become* fat by eating too much food—they actually become fat because *they eat too little.* They consume very calorie-dense foods such as fatty beef, full fat dairy products, and rich desserts that lack the necessary bulk or amount of food to fill them up and satisfy their appetites. As a result, they eat more of the bulk-free foods and end up consuming too many calories. The key to avoiding weight gain is to eat more of the bulky or filling lower calorie foods to begin with. Salads, vegetables, and whole fruits have higher water and lower fat content and are more filling for the calories consumed. Whole grains such as whole wheat bread, brown rice, and whole wheat pasta are also more filling.

Barbara Rolls of the University of Pennsylvania has done some wonderfully convincing studies showing the importance of what she calls the "volumetrics" of weight control. Simply put, if you choose foods with more volume and fewer calories, you will be more successful in controlling your weight or achieving weight loss. Dean Ornish, also a champion of low-fat diets, has written a convincing book entitled *Eat More, Weigh Less.* As an overweight or obese person loses weight, the proper way for him/her to adjust, according to these authorities, is to consume far fewer calories by increasing the *volume or bulk* of the food consumed in order to feel satisfied. Hence eating more to weigh less! And so in a real sense the overweight and obese get fat by eating too little!

How can you take charge and regain control?

For a person to gain weight, his/her average daily **calorie** intake must exceed the average number of calories he/she burns off each day. It may surprise you to know how little that difference really is. Only one hundred extra calories each day will result in a ten-pound weight gain in a year. Now this is actually less of a yearly weight gain than most people generally gain over a lifetime. An annual weight gain of ten pounds would be one hundred pounds in ten years and three hundred pounds in thirty years. Most people who are overweight or even obese do not gain at that rate over the years.

So the healthy change that needs to be made is not that difficult or daunting! Less than one hundred calories a day needs to be eliminated. Of course, averages are deceiving, and someone might gain thirty pounds over a relatively short time with a pregnancy or due to some adverse life event. In most cases, however, the actual daily excess of calories for most people who gain weight over the years is small. One hundred calories is only a pat of butter or less than one tablespoon of oil. Looked at from the aspect of weight loss, one only has to make a few better food choices each week to trim off one hundred calories per day and achieve a ten-pound weight loss (or prevent a ten-pound weight gain) each and every year.

Let's look at some really simple choices someone could make to lose ten pounds in a year (a saving of one hundred calories per day or about seven hundred calories per week):

A small portion of French fries (210 cal) instead of a large portion (540 cal) twice per week (a saving of 330 cal x 2 = 660 cal)

12 oz. diet soda (0 cal) instead of 12 oz. regular soda (150 cal) four to five times per week (a saving of 150 cal x 4-5 = about 700 cal)

One small apple (75 cal) instead of one chocolate bar (235 cal) four to five times per week (a saving of 160 cal x 4-5 = about 700 cal)

One-half cup of Healthy Choice low fat ice cream (110 cal) instead of one-half cup of Häagen-Daz ice cream (330 cal) three to four times per week (a saving of 220 cal x 3-4 = about 700 cal)

6 oz. wild caught salmon (210 cal) instead of 6 oz. rib eye steak (440 cal) three times per week (a saving of 230 cal x 3 = about 700 cal)

These are just a few examples of better food choices for weight control/weight loss. The table on the next page shows many more.

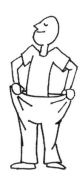

Current Habit [calories]	Try Instead	Calorie saving
1 cup whole milk [150]	1 cup non-fat milk [90]	60

1 oz. regular cheese [110-120]	1 oz. low-fat cheese (e.g. feta or parmesan) [70]	50
4 oz. ground beef (85% lean) [250]	4 oz. ground turkey (85% lean) [180]	70
4 oz. ground beef (85% lean) [250]	4 oz. ground soy "meat" [160]	90
2 eggs [150]	4 egg whites or 1/2 cup egg substitute [60]	90
¼ cup mixed nuts[200]	¼ cup edamame [50]	150
5 oz. wine [100]	5 oz. wine spritzer (2.5 oz. wine + 2.5 oz. sparkling water) [50]	50
4 oz. cream sauce with 1 cup pasta [410]	4 oz. tomato sauce with 1 cup pasta [260]	150
1 cup cream-based soup (cream of broccoli) [205]	1 cup broth-based soup, minestrone [90 calories]	115
2 tbsp. blue cheese dressing [180]	2 tbsp. low-fat blue cheese dressing [80]	100
4 oz. skinless dark chicken meat [230]	4 oz. skinless chicken breast [180]	50
3 oz. tuna salad with 1 tbsp. mayonnaise [200]	3 oz. tuna salad with 1 tbsp. lite mayo (no more than 2 g fat per serving) [125]	75
1 tbsp. regular mayonnaise [100]	1 tbsp. mustard [10] or 1 tbsp. lite mayo [25-50]	90
2 tbsp. tartar sauce [140]	2 tbsp. cocktail sauce [50]	90

5 oz. baked potato w/3 tbsp. sour cream [245]	5 oz. baked potato with ¼ cup salsa + 2 tbsp. non-fat plain yogurt [190]	55
2 tbsp. of oil to sauté (onions, peppers, fish, etc.) [240]	¼ cup broth to sauté (onions, peppers, fish, etc.) or cooking spray [5]	235
1 cup mashed potatoes made with 1 tbsp. butter [235]	1 cup steamed, mixed vegetables with 1 tbsp. lemon juice [80]	155
12 oz. reg. soda [150]	12 oz. diet soda [0]	150
6 oz. low-fat yogurt [180]	6 oz. artificially sweetened non-fat yogurt [90]	90
15 regular tortilla chips [175]	15 baked tortilla chips [125]	50
1 cup orange juice [120]	1 medium orange [65]	55
1 cup orange juice [120]	1 cup tomato juice [50]	70
1 cup grape juice, unsweetened [155]	1 cup grapes [60]	95
½ cup corn or green peas [80]	1 cup steamed broccoli or other non-starchy vegetable [25]	55

Do I Weigh Too Much?

You can calculate your body mass index (BMI) from your weight and height by visiting www.Erectile-Function.com and using the calculator under the Learn More tab or use the table below (if you are between 4 feet 11 inches and 6 feet tall) to see if you weigh enough (considering your height) to be overweight (having a BMI of 25 to 30), obese (a BMI of 30 to 40), or morbidly obese (a BMI of 40 or more):

	Overweight (BMI > 25)	Obese (BMI > 30)	Morbidly obese (BMI > 40)
4 ft. 11 in.	> 123	> 148	> 197
5 ft. 0 in.	> 127	> 153	> 204
5 ft. 1 in.	> 132	> 158	> 211
5 ft. 2 in.	> 136	> 163	> 218
5 ft. 3 in.	> 141	> 169	> 225
5 ft. 4 in.	> 145	> 174	> 232
5 ft. 5 in.	> 150	> 180	> 240
5 ft. 6 in.	> 154	> 185	> 247
5 ft. 7 in.	> 159	> 191	> 255
5 ft. 8 in.	> 164	> 197	> 262
5 ft. 9 in.	> 169	> 203	> 270
5 ft. 10 in.	> 174	> 209	> 278
5 ft. 11 in.	> 179	> 215	> 286
6 ft. 0 in.	> 184	> 221	> 294

Example: If you are five feet four inches and 160 pounds, you are over 145 and therefore overweight, but not over 174, so you are not (yet) obese. A BMI table does not correct for body frame. For someone with a small frame, a rough correction is to subtract 10 percent from the above figures; for a large frame, add 10 percent.

Another very simple calculation that is particularly important for assessing the risk for heart disease and diabetes is the number of inches around your waist, particularly when divided by the number of inches around your hips. Not all fat is equal (or equally bad) and the fat that accumulates around your waistline can be very dangerous. Simply use a tape measure to measure the narrowest part of your middle (if you are unsure, measure at the level of your elbows when your arms are at your sides). Keep the tape snug and parallel to the floor.

For white, black, and Latino men, forty inches or more around the waist signals an increased risk of health problems (thirty-seven inches for Asian men). For white, black, and Latino women, the corresponding figure is thirty-seven inches (thirty-one inches for Asian women).

By measuring the hips at the widest point of your buttocks and dividing the waist measurement by the hip measurement, a ratio of greater than 0.9 for men and 0.8 for women indicates an increased risk of obesity-related disease.

The reason abdominal fat is so important is that it causes insulin resistance. Sugars, alcohol, and simple carbohydrates are deposited preferentially in the abdominal fat (the so-called beer belly). Exercise counters this tendency by increasing the body's sensitivity to insulin.

OK, now that I know that I weigh too much, and that my excess weight may be bad for my erectile health, what other health problems can excess weight cause?

Excess weight is estimated to be responsible for 14 percent of cancer deaths in men and 20 percent in

women. The American Cancer Society has reported that cancers of the breast, colon, rectum, esophagus, liver, gallbladder, pancreas, kidney, uterus, and prostate are related to excess weight, and a study suggested that prostate cancers are more aggressive and are more likely to recur in obese men. Deaths due to non-Hodgkin's lymphoma and multiple myeloma also increase with body weight. Women gaining more than twenty pounds from age eighteen to mid life double their risk of postmenopausal breast cancer compared to women whose weight remains stable.

A weight gain of only eleven to eighteen pounds over normal weight doubles a person's risk of type 2 or adult onset diabetes. A recent study from the Yale School of Public Health predicted that if there is no change in diabetes prevention and care, in twenty years the number of deaths due to diabetes each year in the U.S. will triple to 622,000. And the complications of diabetes such as blindness, limb amputations, and kidney disease will also triple.

For every ten pounds of weight gain there is a 20 percent increase in the likelihood of having high blood pressure. High blood pressure, a poor diet, and diabetes all increase the chance of heart attack and stroke.

A person who is obese has 1.5 times the risk of dying if he or she has a heart attack. Obesity increases abnormal heart rhythms, and both the proliferation of small blood vessels around fat cells and high blood pressure put a strain on the heart at a time when the heart muscle is already starved for blood.

For every two-pound increase in weight, the risk of developing arthritis is increased 9-13 percent. Orthopedic surgeons will tell you that excess body weight is the main cause for hip and knee replacements and that an epidemic of artificial joint surgery is well underway.

For every one unit increase in BMI, Alzheimer's increases 36 percent. A twenty-pound increase of body weight increases BMI about three units, corresponding to over a doubling of the risk of Alzheimer's disease.

Obesity increases gallbladder disease, infertility, urinary incontinence (women), depression, gastro-esophageal reflux disease, macular degeneration of the eye, and pregnancy complications, and any surgery will be much more likely to be complicated in an overweight or obese person. Many physicians say that they would "rather suffer almost any condition besides obesity. At least I would only have to deal with a single disease instead of a whole multitude of health problems that accompany obesity."

So how do I go about losing weight?

Lasting weight loss requires fundamental changes in eating behavior and physical activity levels. You must make healthier choices that are permanent. For example, many people could solve their weight problem by cutting out all fried foods. The calories in oil are extremely concentrated, and frying may actually add up to several hundred calories to a meal. In the case of French fries, partially hydrogenated oils are usually used. Partially hydrogenated oils contain trans fats, which are worse than saturated fat and are strongly linked to heart disease. Trans fats have twice the adverse impact of saturated fat on the LDL/HDL cholesterol ratio. It has been estimated that trans fats are responsible for between 30,000 and 100,000 premature deaths from heart disease each year in the U.S. An increase of 2 percent of total calories from trans fat has been linked to a 40 percent increase of type 2 or adult-onset diabetes.

Research has found that lasting weight loss is linked to lower fat intake and increased physical activity. A thirty-minute walk at least five days per week will trim about one hundred calories per day and ten pounds in a year. If you walk for an hour every day, that alone will lead to a twenty-five-pound weight loss in a year. If you do weight training, the increased muscle mass will burn off calories even when you are at rest (muscle tissue is more metabolically active than fat tissue and will burn more calories even at rest).

Eat regular meals, monitor your weight, and be consistent in your weight control behaviors. The idea that you can "take a holiday" from good eating habits at parties or on the weekend will set you up for failure.

Here are some easy steps to take:

> ➤ Make changes in eating habits and activity that will together trim at least three hundred calories per day (see the expanded electronic book available for download at no extra charge online for examples of changes you can make).

> ➤ Commit to these two changes above and incorporate them into your daily routine. After a month, the changes will become positive habits.

> ➤ After one month, identify the next new changes and repeat the process. Make sure that you continue the previous changes. Trimming five hundred calories per day should result in a one-pound weight loss per week (fifty pounds per year—see "Some simple calculations"). We do not suggest trimming more than a total of one thousand calories per day (two pounds weight loss per week), and

in general we suggest gradual weight reduction (twenty to thirty pounds per year) to minimize the slowing of metabolism that goes along with more severe calorie restriction. We recommend three servings of dairy daily (1,200 mg of calcium daily) because of the positive effects of calcium and dairy proteins in accelerating weight loss.

What other things can I do to help me lose weight?

Eat a good breakfast and avoid sweets and simple carbohydrates that are rapidly absorbed as sugar and stimulate your insulin levels. A recent study showed that people who skip breakfast consume on average one hundred more calories per day. That will cause a weight gain of one hundred pounds in ten years, so this factor alone can cause a person to become obese. When you skip breakfast and then have a sugary snack such as doughnuts or a Danish pastry (both also loaded with trans fats), your blood sugar and insulin levels will soar followed by low blood sugar, making you famished for lunch, at which time you overeat.

This cycle can continue all day, with each spike in insulin making you excessively hungry for the next meal or snack. Spreading out your intake of energy and keeping your blood sugar lower and more even will help to control your appetite. Also, sugar in excessive amounts is bad for blood vessel health. The only difference between a juvenile diabetic and a healthy person is generally higher levels of blood sugar, and over many years these individuals can develop very serious cardiovascular problems, in part because high blood sugar interferes with NO production by the lining of blood vessels.

Get a good night's sleep. A recent study showed that compared with people getting seven to eight hours of sleep, an average of only six hours of sleep increased obesity by about 20 percent, five hours of sleep by 50 percent, and less than four hours of sleep by about 75 percent. These shorter sleep durations are associated with reduced levels of leptin, a substance in the blood that blunts appetite, and increased blood levels of ghrelin, which stimulates our appetite.

Buffets and parties encourage overeating because of the profusion of food available. Spoil your appetite before you go by having an apple or some low-fat yogurt. You don't have to try everything. Pick only a few things that really appeal to you and hopefully are nutritious and not full of fat or sugar. If you have a serious weight problem, avoid buffets, and the last place on earth you should go for a vacation is an all-inclusive (i.e. all you can eat) resort.

Eat slowly to allow yourself to feel full. Enjoying food with good company will slow you down. Stop before you feel full and either leave the rest on your plate or take it home. You will save much more money by not becoming obese than you could ever lose by leaving food uneaten.

When shopping, look closely at nutrition labels. The number of calories can be deceiving—the portion size is often less than you will be eating. For example, a frozen pizza may list the calorie content as 330 calories per serving, which sounds reasonable. However, when you then look at "number of servings per container" it might say "8." That means if you will be satisfied with one slice, it might be considered a reasonable choice if you are watching your weight. However, if you know you will probably eat half of the pizza you would then have to multiply the 330 calories by four for a total calorie content of 1,320! The amount of fat should not be greater than three grams per hundred calories (3 grams of fat at 9 cal per gram = 27 calories or 27 percent of the 100 calories). Overall we recommend that you consume 20-25 percent of your calories as fat. Provided you limit individual foods to no more than 27 percent of calories (3 grams per 100 calories), your average will be in the right range, since many other foods will be lower.

Beware of eating out. You have little control over calorie and fat content of foods in restaurants and fast-food outlets, so find out as much as you can before going. Most fast-food outlets post nutritional information on their websites. A salad might sound like a good choice, but the standard dressing can add major calories and fat. For a hamburger, the difference between adding mustard and ketchup instead of their special dressing could be one hundred calories or more. Pick restaurants you know offer more healthy fare, share an entrée or dessert, have them bring the bread with the main course, and take food home rather than finishing everything on your plate. The expanded book, which is available for download online, has more suggestions for "healthy eating out."

Avoid all sugary sodas, power drinks, fruit juices, and coffee drinks spiked with calories. A recent large study showed that consuming at least one sugar-sweetened soft drink per day almost doubled the risk of type 2 diabetes. A far better choice than fruit juice is a piece of whole fruit. It has fewer calories, more bulk and fiber, and the skin has the largest amount of antioxidants. Note that some specialty coffees can have up to 600 calories, 24 grams of fat, 14 grams of saturated fat, and 70 grams of sugar! After adding real whipping cream on top (another 100 calories), a simple cup of coffee can end up having as many calories as a very large lunch! Try having only the coffee and you'll be surprised how much you will appreciate the taste of the coffee itself.

If you are really serious about losing weight, avoid alcohol. Alcohol is very calorie-dense (7 calories per gram), is more rapidly absorbed than carbohydrates, and promotes fat deposition in the abdominal area. Most drinks are 100 to 200 calories (wine is about 90 calories for 4 oz., beer is close to 120 calories for 12 oz., and mixed drinks are 150 to 300 calories depending on mixers), so an extra drink or two adds significant calories.

Avoid fatty beef or pork: Beef can vary from quite lean to as much as 30-40 percent fat. *Time* magazine cited an example of classic baby back ribs with 1,437 calories and 92 grams of fat (828 calories just from the fat). If you must have red meat, there are lots of lean cuts that have only slightly more saturated fat than chicken (e.g. top round, top sirloin steak, or round tip roast). At the very least, trim off any fat before cooking. Ground beef generally comes in various percentages of fat. We have found that 15 percent is a reasonable compromise between taste and unnecessary calories.

Avoid rich desserts: A dessert with a lot of fat and sugar can contain 500 to as much as 1,000 calories. If you have to lose a lot of weight, don't go there at all. Or else take a very small serving and savor each bite. A common suggestion is to try only three bites and stop. Forego real whipped cream or push it off to the side. Instead, try berries or a scoop of healthy ice cream like Healthy Choice. These "smarter" ice creams can be incredibly good and contain as little as 110 calories per scoop and only 1.5 grams of fat.

Choose tomato or lemon-based sauces instead of a creamy sauce: You'll trim a couple of hundred calories right there and you will also avoid the unhealthy saturated fat in the cream.

Avoid all deep-fried foods: A tablespoon of oil is 120 calories. Anything deep-fried can have one hundred to several hundred calories sticking to it or absorbed by it. Even pan frying can add a lot of oil. Watch out for things like eggplant, which can sop up a surprising quantity of calorie-containing oil.

Shopping hints for buying foods with the same volume but fewer calories (You're going to be eating what you buy, so the right choices *start here*):

➤ It's best not to shop when you're really hungry and to prepare a list of items rather than picking up anything that looks tempting.

➤ Shop in stores that place more emphasis on healthy alternatives, such as Trader Joe's or Whole Foods.

➤ Yogurt can have over 200 calories for 8 ounces or as few as 100 calories with no fat if you choose a non-fat fruit-flavored version with an artificial sweetener (e.g. Kroger brand Lite Yogurt).

➤ Some white cheeses such as mozzarella, goat, feta, or lite Jarlsberg cheese (if made from part-skim milk) will have fewer calories and fat than cheeses made from whole fat milk. Feta cheese is a particularly good choice when used in moderation since it has lots of flavor and only 60 calories and 4 grams of fat per one-ounce serving. Mozzarella or "string cheese" is another good low-calorie cheese for an easy snack. Grated parmesan, romano, or pecorino cheeses are also a good source of flavor without a lot of fat or calories.

➤ Nulaid Reddi Egg or other real egg substitutes have only 30 calories and 0 grams of fat per serving (1/4 cup = 1 whole egg) and make delicious scrambled eggs and omelets, whereas a regular fresh whole egg has 80 calories and 5 grams of fat. Adding fresh tomatoes, salsa, spinach, mushrooms, onions, and small amounts of low- or non-fat cheese can help you create tasty breakfasts without adding lots of calories and fat.

➢ One of the best products we have found as a spread for toast is Brummel & Brown spread, which is 35 percent vegetable oil and 10 percent yogurt. With only 45 calories per tablespoon and 5 grams of fat, this product tastes as good or better than other spreads on the market with about half the calories and fat. It also has minimal trans fatty acids and no cholesterol per serving. Smart Balance is a similar product that can be used for cooking.

➢ Kraft makes a very flavorful "Lite Mayo" with 45 calories per tablespoon and only 4 grams of fat. "Just 2 Good" is another lite mayo with only 25 calories and 2 grams of fat. We like to make our own lite mayo/chipotle chile spread by adding canned chipotle chiles in adobo sauce to the lite mayo. Since this spread is quite hot you need very little chipotle mayo to add lots of flavor to a sandwich or tuna or egg salad.

➢ When it comes to breakfast and lunch meats, avoid salami, pastrami, and other high-fat deli meats. Lean turkey and chicken lunch meats and even turkey pastrami and turkey ham are much better choices. If you are a bacon and sausage lover try Morningstar Farms brand soy protein-based bacon and breakfast sausage. They are both very low in fat and calories and have lots of flavor and good texture. Trader Joe's has a great low-fat chicken sausage in their deli section. If you want real bacon, be sure to choose Canadian bacon, which has far less fat.

> ➢ Ice creams and sorbets are examples of dessert treats that can be fairly healthy or incredibly unhealthy. Again, it's all about reading and understanding labels. One popular brand of rich ice cream features flavors ranging from 180 to 310 calories and 10 to 21 grams of fat per ½-cup serving. In contrast, Healthy Choice makes a very creamy and delicious low-fat ice cream line with as little as 110 calories and 1.5 grams of fat per ½-cup serving.

One of the great paradoxes of this decade is that we have never had as many great food products to help us reduce calorie intake, nor as much information showing the extensive health risks of obesity. And yet we have never had as many overweight people. We hope this book and the expanded version available for download online will bridge this information gap and provide the knowledge and simple methods needed to make lasting changes in your eating habits.

In most cases, a change in food preferences is required before the unwanted pounds can melt away. If you have become accustomed to deriving flavor from high fat and high sugar, you may think that changing to other sources of flavor will not be enjoyable. Be assured that your tastes will change and you will learn to like the new flavors as much or more. How many of us have switched from regular milk to nonfat milk? Initially the nonfat version tasted "watery," and we missed the "mouth feel" of the fat in the whole milk. But after a few weeks (perhaps as few as three weeks), the nonfat version became actually palatable and the whole-fat milk seemed too rich and thick (somewhat like cream). We learned to prefer the nonfat version because it was what we drank regularly.

You will actually get to the point that high fat and high sugar no longer taste as good as you remembered. Also, your digestive tract will change so that you feel uncomfortable with a higher fat intake. We're not saying that you will never enjoy dessert again. But you will probably get even more enjoyment from a dessert that is less sweet and lower in fat than you are now accustomed to. You will also enjoy the healthier food more because you will know you're doing something positive rather than negative for your health, just as you enjoy food more with good company.

If your attitude is "if it's good for me it will taste bad," then give us a chance to change your perception of the taste of healthy foods. Try a few of our recipes (available online at www.Erectile-Function.com). We'll show you how to make changes so that you are not disappointed with the new flavors and textures inherent in healthier foods. We'll give you some examples so you will learn to modify some of your favorite recipes to lower the fat and sugar content and to increase the fiber and water content to increase satiety.

Everybody's Doing it – It Must be OK

People can be very much like sheep or birds flying in formation. They may feel most comfortable following others rather than making the mental effort to decide which direction to go themselves. The problem is that sometimes the leader or the crowd is going in the wrong direction. At Enron, for instance, it became the corporate norm to follow business practices that were illegal, and people followed others to personal disaster.

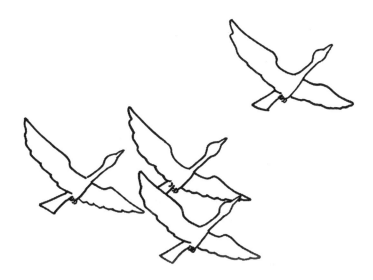

Choose those that you follow carefully!

If two-thirds of people are overweight, it can't be that bad, can it? If everyone is eating French fries, doughnuts and Danish pastries, all full of trans fats, it can't be that bad, can it? If the Atkin's diet is a best-seller, it can't be that bad, can it?

Well, actually, the simple fact is that when it comes to nutrition and weight control, if you follow the crowd, you could be in for some very nasty surprises. It *can* be that bad.

Some of the Scientific Evidence Supporting this Chapter:

1) de Kreutzenberg SV, et al.: Elevated non-esterified fatty acids impair nitric oxide independent vasodilation in humans. Atherosclerosis. 2003;169:147-53

2) Bray, GA: Obesity is a chronic, relapsing neurochemical disease. Int J Obes Relat Metab Disord. 2004;28:34-8

3) Esposito K, et al.: Effect of lifestyle changes on erectile dysfunction in obese men: a randomized controlled study. JAMA 2004;291:2978-84

4) Welborn TA, et al.: Waist-hip ratio is the dominant factor predicting cardiovascular death in Australia. Med J Aust 2003;179:580-5

Chapter Three

Failure to Firm Up – Medical Causes of ED

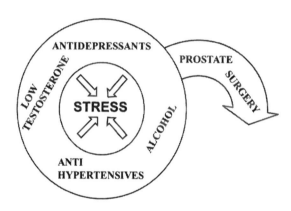

Erectile dysfunction, or ED (also known as impotence), is the inability to achieve or to maintain a firm erection that is sufficient for sexual intercourse, ejaculation, or both. It occurs to some degree in a little more than half of men between the ages forty and seventy, with the number of men affected rising from about four out of ten by age forty to nearly seven out of ten by the age of seventy. Not too many years ago it was assumed that almost all of the cases of ED were caused by psychological problems such as anxiety or depression. Today experts agree that about nine out of every ten men with ED have medical or physical causes and that few men with ED have psychological problems alone as the cause of their poor erectile health.

The penis has two parallel columns of spongy tissue called the corpora cavernosa, or erectile bodies. A third middle chamber called the corpus spongiosum contains the urethra or tube that carries urine from the bladder through the penis and out of the body during urination. This tube also carries sperm and seminal fluid, the ejaculate, from the testicles and prostate gland during male orgasm. The erectile tissues of the penis contain tiny pools of blood vessels known as cavernous sinuses. Smooth muscle and elastic tissue called collagen surround the cavernous sinuses.

Most of the time, the penis is "resting" and non-erect. This normally changes quickly when a state of sexual arousal occurs. In the non-erect state the small blood vessels leading to the cavernous sinuses contract and become narrow, reducing the flow of blood into the penis. During sexual arousal the male central nervous system stimulates the release of several chemicals including nitric oxide (NO), which is considered the major chemical that begins and maintains a firm erection. NO then stimulates the production of cyclic GMP (see chapter one), the chemical that relaxes the smooth muscle in the penis, allowing blood to flow into the penis. This flooding of blood into the penis nearly doubles its diameter, squeezing the veins around the chambers and preventing the blood from draining out. The penis becomes firm, rigid, and erect. Fairly soon after ejaculation, cyclic GMP is broken down by the enzyme PDE_5, causing the penis to return to its non-erect state.

A proper balance of body gases, chemicals, and other substances are very important for erectile health and sexual function. Two of the most important are oxygen and collagen (connective tissue). Oxygen-rich blood is necessary for erectile health. We all might want to think about this fact the next time we are in a smoke-filled room or a smoggy city! Oxygen suppresses an immune system growth factor in smooth muscle called a cytokine that can cause too much collagen to form in the corpora cavernosa of the penis. This can contribute to ED. Oxygen also helps erectile health by increasing the activity of prostaglandin E1, which reduces collagen production (a good thing) and promotes the release of calcium in smooth muscle, allowing relaxation and increased blood flow into the penis.

Although ED is more common as most men age, it does not have to be an inevitable consequence of getting older. The effect of age on erectile health has more to do with several diseases and conditions such as heart disease, diabetes, and hypertension (high blood pressure), which are more common in older men. The good news is that these physical causes of ED along with a few other conditions that may occur with age are avoidable in some cases and controllable most of the time. We now know that erectile health can be improved by natural methods and medication when necessary—more about this later.

Before going over the medical and physical conditions that can cause ED, there are a few lifestyle and psychological causes that should be mentioned. Excessive anxiety and depression can cause ED. Anxiety and concern about sexual performance can result in the release of substances that cause blood vessels to narrow and prevent blood flow into the penis. Depression is strongly associated with ED with at least eight out of ten depressed men in one study reporting moderate to severe ED. Depression also reduces sexual desire, although it is not always clear which is the cause and which is the effect.

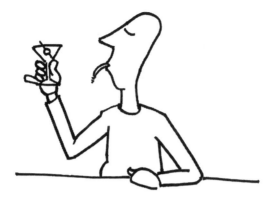

Smoking and excessive use of alcohol are the two most preventable causes of ED. Smoking harms blood vessels, leading to high blood pressure and atherosclerosis, or hardening of the arteries, that can cause ED. Ever wonder why the Marlboro Man was always alone in those commercials? Even though small amounts of alcohol may release inhibitions and promote sexual activity, more than one ounce of alcohol (one carefully poured drink) in most men depresses the central nervous system and harms erectile performance.

Several highly preventable medical conditions aggravate the biggest problem leading to ED—unhealthy blood vessels that fail to open and allow blood flow into the penis. These conditions include diabetes, heart disease, hypertension (high blood pressure), and blood vessel disease of the extremities. Obesity, poor nutrition, lack of exercise, and unhealthy lifestyle choices such as smoking and excessive use of alcohol worsen these diseases. NO, the major substance responsible for good erectile health, is reduced in all of these conditions.

Some experts believe that diabetes alone is responsible for over 40 percent of ED. The chronically higher levels of blood sugar decrease NO production from the lining of blood vessels. Dr. Louis Ignarro, who wrote the foreword in this book, was awarded the Nobel Prize in medicine in 1998. He and his team at the David Geffen School of Medicine at UCLA have shown that the excess sugar in the blood of those with diabetes combines with low density lipoproteins (LDL—the bad type of lipoprotein cholesterol), reducing the blood vessel production of NO. Nerve damage is also common in diabetics and this may also lead to ED.

Heart disease, the leading cause of death in men and women in the U.S., is very often associated with ED. One recent study showed that increased levels of an amino acid called homocysteine can predict the risk of ED. Homocysteine is elevated in men who go on to develop heart disease and stroke and is decreased by folic acid supplementation. ED is frequently reported by men who have high blood pressure. In fact, nearly half of men with ED also have elevated blood pressure. In part this relationship occurs because obesity, poor diet, and inactivity contribute to both conditions and, in part, because the hardening and narrowing of the arteries resulting from the high blood pressure reduces blood flow through the penile arteries. Unfortunately many of the medicines that are used to treat hypertension can cause ED. The newer drugs used to treat high blood pressure, such as angiotensin-converting enzyme (ACE) inhibitors and angiotensin-receptor blockers (ARBs), are less likely to cause ED. Recent studies show that ARBs may actually restore erectile health in men with high blood pressure and ED.

Several other less common medical conditions and diseases that can disturb erectile health include Parkinson's disease, multiple sclerosis (MS), and epilepsy. Impaired nerve function probably explains why men with these medical problems frequently have ED. A few more common conditions such as allergies, thyroid and lung disease have been linked to ED. It is not totally clear, however, how these more common diseases cause ED.

Surgery for prostate cancer and prostate cancer itself can cause ED by damaging the nerves necessary for healthy erectile function. Even radiation therapy that may be used to treat prostate cancer can cause ED, although to a lesser extent than radical prostatectomy (surgical removal of the prostate gland and surrounding tissues). Some of the newer nerve-sparing procedures are reported to result in less ED.

Most of the chronic conditions and diseases mentioned above can be prevented or improved by controlling weight, being active, and following a nutritious diet. Even the development of prostate cancer is significantly reduced by avoiding obesity and maintaining optimum nutrition. So be firm about eating well. Continue or start to exercise to become firm and you should stay firm longer!

Chapter Four

en Nature Needs Help –
atment Choices for ED

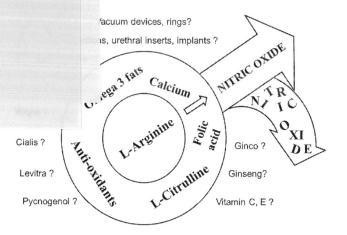

Keep in mind that no matter what therapy is used to treat ED, establishing a healthy lifestyle should be the first and most important step for maintaining and restoring erectile health. Before any treatment for ED is begun, all options should be reviewed with the help of your physician and the involvement of your sexual partner. Any medical conditions you may have should be reviewed and the likely benefit and safety of any potential treatment considered. Because some of the options involve untested and unregulated substances, the risk of harm from the treatment may not be completely known. Also, some options involve the use of devices and injections that may reduce spontaneity, lowering the comfort level and satisfaction for both you and your sexual partner. Treatment options for ED include natural substances, prescription oral medications, injections, topical medications, blood flow devices, and penile implants.

Natural Substances

In addition to omega-3, antioxidant, calcium, and folic acid supplementation (covered in the introduction) several herbal remedies have been identified as helpful for maintaining and restoring erectile health (see Chapter Seven – "Supplements for Erectile Health"). They are thought to work by improving blood flow and increasing the production of NO. Yohimbine, also known as Yocon or Yohimex, is available without prescription and has been recommended in a dose range of 5 to 10 mg by some experts, although the American Urological Society does not recommend it for ED because of a lack of reliable information on its safety and efficacy. Yohimbine has been used in combination with L-arginine, the amino acid from which NO is produced. There have been concerns regarding the safety of Yohimbine. In two studies L-arginine appeared to be of some help, but in other studies there was no apparent benefit. Taking L-arginine may be important if a person's intake of protein is reduced.

Other Asian herbal remedies such as ginseng and gingko are widely used in some parts of the world to improve sexual performance. It is important to remember that studies that measure the effectiveness and safety of these herbal remedies are either not available because they have not been done or have confusing results. It is also important to keep in mind that these supplements are not evaluated as carefully by government regulators. In one study, measureable levels of sildenafil, vardenafil, or tadalafil (the active ingredients in the Viagra-like drugs) were found in nearly half of the supplements that were tested. The amounts varied, and there is no way to know how much is contained in these products. This is one of the reasons these herbal chemicals and supplements should never be used without the supervision of a medical professional. Even small amounts of Viagra-like medications can have serious side effects or even be fatal when taken in combination with certain medicines, particularly nitroglycerin.

Prescription Oral Medications

CAUTION: be **very careful** when using Viagra-like drugs after optimizing your NO production following the recommendations on our website or in our books. You could have an exaggerated response with a very prolonged erection (called priapism) that can require a trip to the emergency room. We recommend that you carefully read and follow the precautions in the package insert and start with one-quarter of the lowest dose and gradually increase once you know you are not having this problem. You should expect to respond to lower doses of these drugs—and at least you will spend less and get more pleasure from using these drugs if you need them.

There are currently three Food and Drug Administration (FDA)-approved prescription oral medications for

the treatment of ED. The first drug approved was sildenafil, or Viagra, the most known and widely used. Viagra
belongs to a group of drugs that block the enzyme PDE5
that breaks down cyclic GMP, allowing enough cyclic GMP
to accumulate and relax the smooth muscle in the penis
(see chapter one). This relaxation allows for the increased
blood flow into the penis that results in a firm erection.
Two other oral prescription medications are now available
that work the way Viagra does but are longer acting—vardenafil (Levitra) and tadalafil (Cialis).

All three selective enzyme inhibitors have been studied
and approved by the FDA to be safe and effective for the
treatment of ED. These prescription medications do have
side-effects and complications, however. Recently blindness
that may be related to use of these medications has been
reported in very rare instances. These drugs should never
be used without close medical supervision. Side-effects and
complications of all medications are usually less severe or
do not occur with lower doses. Beginning and maintaining a healthy lifestyle (proper diet and adequate exercise)
may allow for the use of a lower dose of these medications
if and when they are needed to treat ED. The lowest necessary dose is always the safest way to use any drug.

Injections and Topical Medications

The oral prescription medications may not be safe or
effective for everyone because of underlying health problems. They also do not work for everyone with ED. Penile
injections of medications such as phentolamine, alprosta-
dil, or papaverine can be very effective for ED. Alprosta-
dil is derived from prostaglandin E1, a natural substance,
and works by increasing blood flow into the penis. Medications that are injected into the penis (products such as

Caverject or Edex), delivered into the urethra—the urine tube in the middle of the penis—(the MUSE system), and topical creams (products such as Alprox-TD and Topiglan) are available. These products require a prescription and supervision by medical professionals.

Blood Flow Devices

Several devices are available for the treatment of ED. Vacuum devices and non-vacuum venous flow systems are reasonably simple to use and are safe and effective. To use the vacuum device the man inserts his penis into a plastic cylinder. When a vacuum is created inside this cylinder blood flows into the penis and a firm erection occurs. An elastic band is placed around the base of the penis to maintain the erection and the penis is removed from the cylinder. Because it takes up to five minutes to produce a firm erection, this method may interfere with spontaneity and be unacceptable to some. Men who have erections but have difficulty maintaining one can use a ring placed at the base of the penis (such as Actis) to prevent blood from escaping from an already erect penis. These devices should not be used for more than thirty minutes each time because they block needed oxygen to the penis.

Penile Implants

Surgical implants are available for men who may fail other less invasive treatments for ED. Nearly a quarter of a million of these procedures were performed during the 1980s with good results and high satisfaction. Some implants are always "erect" and others are inflatable. However, these options have become less popular with the introduction of effective oral prescription medications.

Prevention of ED

Erectile health can now be protected to a greater extent during surgery for prostate cancer. The prostatectomy (removal of the prostate gland) is performed in a way designed to avoid injury to the nerves and blood vessels that are most important for erectile function. This approach is not always successful, but men who elect to have surgery for prostate cancer respond well to many of the other options for treating ED that have already been mentioned.

Benjamin Franklin, one of our founding fathers and a man who lived into his ninth decade, once said that "an ounce of prevention is worth a pound of cure." There is no way to know for sure if Mr. Franklin was speaking from personal experience about firmness. However, he was known as a ladies' man late into his life, traveled frequently to Paris, and was said to always have a twinkle in his eye! One wonders whether preservation of his erectile health had anything to do with his longevity and his outlook on life. It is doubtful that he knew about Omega-3s or folic acid, but he did live in Philadelphia, a port city near the ocean with an abundance of seafood.

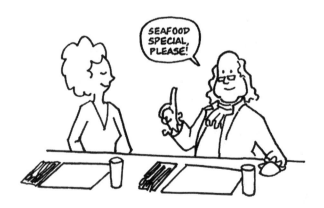

The Future of ED treatment: It may be possible to someday reverse ED by gene therapy. Dr. Louis Ignarro's team has shown that NO production can be increased by injecting a gene for NO synthesis directly into the penile tissue. Such an effect would be permanent rather than the temporary effect of other penile injections. So even if everything discussed in this book and the excellent drugs available for treating ED are not effective, the future still may hold real promise.

Some of the Scientific Evidence Supporting this Chapter

1) Champion HC, Bivalacqua TJ, Hyman AL, Ignarro LJ, Hellstrom WJ, Kadowitz PJ: Gene transfer of endothelial nitric oxide synthase to the penis augments erectile responses in the aged rat. Proc Natl Acad Sci USA. 1999;96:13-52.

Chapter Five

Good Blood Flow –
A Good Pump and Good Pipes Too

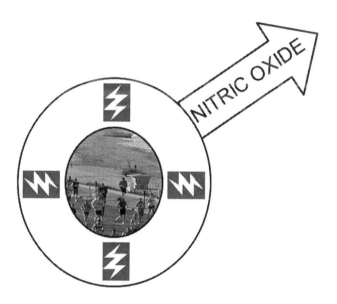

An adequate erection will occur when a large amount of blood fills the penis and stays there. And all of this blood is needed at the same time that the heart and blood vessels must supply other parts of the body that also need blood during love-making. It is estimated that intercourse can consume as many as seven hundred calories per hour, which is equivalent to a very vigorous physical workout!

Someone who does not exercise regularly will likely have a heart and blood vessels that are unprepared and unable to respond to this increased demand for blood flow. It should not be surprising that ED is linked strongly to physical inactivity. Men who do not exercise regularly are Two to ten times more likely to have ED. The hopeful news is that the Massachusetts Male Aging Study found that a brisk daily walk reduced the likelihood of ED by 70 percent. Other research has found that moderate physical activity reduced the risk of ED by two-thirds and in men with high physical activity, the ED risk was reduced by over 80%!

But why does this regular physical activity help so much? Many studies have shown that exercise increases NO production in the lining cells (endothelium) of blood vessels. This very likely explains the well-known beneficial effects of exercise on the heart and blood vessels and on erectile health. Physical activity also improves the good kind of cholesterol (HDL) and lowers blood sugar by improving the way the body uses insulin. So it is not just your heart that benefits from exercise: another organ between your legs benefits too! You will also feel better in general and be able to enjoy both outdoor and indoor physical activities. Exercise is also the best way to trim excess abdominal fat. Your partner may rediscover those hidden love handles that she used to be able to hold onto.

Our bodies use energy or calories in two major ways. First, the energy is used to maintain our basal metabolism (the involuntary activities necessary to keep us alive, such as our heart beat and body temperature). This is often referred to as our basal metabolic rate, or BMR. And second, energy is used for voluntary physical activity (the intentional activities that we do, such as walking, running, and swimming.)

A person's BMR is somewhat individual and not everyone uses calories at the same rate. When the average person consumes 2,000 calories each day, 60-70 percent of those calories, or about 1,300 calories per day, are used to support their involuntary activities or basal metabolism. An individual's BMR usually declines with age due to a decrease in lean body mass (muscle and non-fatty tissue). However, research has shown that if we maintain lean body mass with exercise, we can prevent or at least decrease this decline in BMR. Physical activity such as strength training (with weights or other forms of resistance) helps to preserve the lean body mass, or muscle structure. As little as a half hour two to three times per week spent exercising muscle groups can preserve our muscle mass and enhance our ability to burn more calories.

Differences in BMR may be genetic. For example, the high rate of obesity among African American women over the age of forty may be due in large part to a genetically programmed BMR that is 5 percent lower than Caucasian women. Unfortunately this makes weight control more challenging for these women. This 5 percent difference amounts to about sixty-five calories less per day that they can eat or that they will have to burn through exercise just to make up for their lower BMR.

The CDC now recommends thirty minutes of moderate exercise most days of the week. If you combine this with twice-weekly weight training, your muscles will burn more calories even when you're at rest.

We can have the most control over our energy use by adjusting the amount of physical activity such as by walking, running, playing tennis, or doing any number of other activities that require voluntary physical exertion. Just as you can easily shave off a couple of hundred calories from your diet by making better food choices, you can easily expend an extra hundred or two hundred calories each day by being more physically active. Although it is a bit easier to trim calories by reducing food intake than by burning them off through exercise, doing both is the winning combination. Regular exercise also increases an important antioxidant that is lower in men with ED. When combined with strength training, the extra muscle becomes more metabolically active, resulting in a higher BMR and more calories burned.

The number of calories expended with any type of exercise varies with weight. Our website gives a simple way to calculate the number of calories you will burn with various activities corrected for your body weight. Be sure to check with your physician before embarking on any new program of physical exercise.

Sounds good – so how much should I do?

The Centers for Disease Control (CDC) currently recommends 30 minutes of moderate activity most days of the week. Estimating 150 calories for moderate physical activity during five days per week you would burn 750 calories, or approximately 100 calories per day. Combine this with trimming 200 calories from your diet and you can turn a weight gain of 10 pounds per year into a 20 pound weight loss per year. The expanded book that is available for download online has more information about how to calculate various strategies to lose and control your weight.

Some may prefer to do an hour of strenuous exercise twice per week, again averaging a little over 100 calories per day. Although it is probably best to spread it more evenly throughout the week as the CDC recommends for overall health benefits, more strenuous cardiovascular fitness may be the way to go for erectile firmness.

In addition to the physical activities that most people call exercise, you can burn a significant number of calories by getting up and moving whenever the opportunity presents itself. We call this "exercise in real-time," which means physically moving at home or on the job—whenever possible each day—to increase your physical activity level without taking extra time. This can decrease the special time needed for regular exercise. If your office is on the second or third floor, take the stairs. Instead of using the telephone or e-mail, make a personal visit to discuss an issue with someone else in the office. On the way home from work when you stop to do an errand, take the first parking place you see, rather than circling around until you find a place closest to the entrance. When you come back to your car from shopping, leave the cart at the store exit and carry your purchases to the car.

Whenever possible, stand rather than sit and you will burn more calories. Carry your luggage rather than pulling it on rollers. Even Bill Gates, one of the richest men in the world, carries his own luggage. If you take advantage of every opportunity to expend a few extra calories, it can easily amount to fifty calories per day, which will amount to another five pounds of weight loss per year!

Take the stairs instead of the elevator, take the first parking spot (not the closest) you see when running an errand, leave the grocery cart at the store entrance, and walk to any destination less than a mile away. You are decreasing our reliance on oil imports and saving wear and tear on your car while improving your health at the same time.

A pedometer will give you a helpful measure of your activity, and a goal to aim for (at least 10,000 steps per day).

It can be very helpful to have some measure of your physical activity that you can use to set goals. Pedometers are inexpensive step-counters that allow you to keep track of your total daily activity. They are very accurate when used at a moderate pace, such as three miles per hour. For people who walk more slowly, a piezoelectric device will be more suitable. The recommended minimum for optimal health is 10,000 steps per day. Using a pedometer is a good way to get an idea of how much movement you are currently doing and how much you need to increase. James O. Hill, PhD, has popularized the pedometer in a book called *The Step Diet Book: Count Steps, Not Calories to Lose Weight and Keep It Off Forever*, which comes with a pedometer. The book clearly emphasizes his research findings that long-term success in weight loss depends on reducing calories *and* moving more.

Can I just exercise and not worry about my weight?

Ignoring weight loss and only exercising may be tempting. A recent study, however, showed a 30 percent increase in mortality for people who were overweight and fit as well as in those who were normal weight and were unfit, compared with a 50-60 percent increase in people who were both overweight and unfit. Fitness may reduce the risk of death, even without weight loss, but not to the same extent as when exercise is combined with weight loss.

> *Choose exercise you enjoy and do it with friends. You will be more likely to make exercise a habit for life.*

Exercising with friends or people with common interests is more enjoyable, and you will be more likely to stick with an exercise program. Walk with a friend and you will save time by combining a social visit with the exercise. Think back to the things you've enjoyed doing in the past. You might want to buy a bicycle or take up golf again. If you enjoy hiking, join the Sierra Club, or other similar types of walking and hiking groups, and you may make new friends who also value exercise and good health. Get a friend to follow the recommendations in this book and have the pleasure of seeing that person become healthier together with you. A healthy life style can be fun!

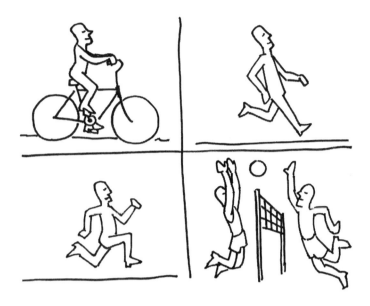

Considering all of the options for exercise and weight loss mentioned, it is likely that exercises aimed at cardiovascular fitness, such as jogging or using an elliptical trainer, will give you the best results for improving your love life. Vigorous exercise over short periods of time such as thirty to sixty minutes also increases testosterone levels. Just remember, if you get short of breath walking up one flight of stairs, it is a sign that your heart is unable to keep up with this modest demand for increased blood flow. When you are having sex, you are exercising and at the same time your erection is requiring a thirty- to forty-fold increase in blood flow to the penis. If you are obese, the numerous small blood vessels around your fat cells are also drawing away blood. Good sexual performance requires you to be in good shape, and the fact that you look better and sexier may provide more opportunities for good sex!

Chapter Six

Good Nutrition Makes for Good Sex

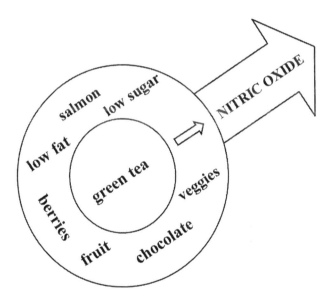

The link between good nutrition and healthy erections is well established. We know, for example, that omega-3 fats, folic acid, antioxidants, and calcium all help to stimulate the production of NO, the main initiator (besides sexual stimuli, of course) of an erection. The amount of these nutrients is usually not sufficient, however, in the diet of the general population in the U.S. This leads to more heart and blood vessel disease and cancer. These important nutrients have many other health benefits in addition to better erections, as you will see.

Omega-3 Fatty Acids:

Omega-3 fatty acids decrease heart attacks, irregular heart rhythms that can lead to sudden death, and stroke. They reduce blood clotting and the level of triglycerides (harmful fats) in the blood, may lower blood pressure somewhat, and may reduce inflammation in blood vessel walls, a key cause of blood vessel blockage that triggers heart attacks and strokes. There is also some evidence that they decrease colon and prostate cancer, and some studies Have shown a lower incidence of depression. Omega-3 and omega-6 fatty acids are called essential because the body cannot make enough of them. They must therefore be supplied by the diet or by supplementation.

The two most important types of omega-3 fatty acids are EPA, or eicosapentaenoic acid, and DHA, or docosahexaenoic acid. The typical Western diet that most Americans eat has ample amounts of omega-6 fatty acids; however, it usually does not contain enough omega-3 fatty acids. The omega-6 fatty acids are found in oils made from corn, sunflower, safflower, and soybean and in meats such as beef and poultry. Health experts estimate that the typical American diet has far too much omega-6 fat compared to omega-3 fat. It can be healthy to consume more omega-6 fats than omega-3 fats, but omega-3s should be at least one-third of the total amount of these essential fats in the diet (www.consumerlabs.com).

In order to obtain the right balance between omega-3 and omega-6 fatty acids, most of us should eat more fish and less red meat and poultry. Three and a half ounces of fatty fish such as salmon, sardines, anchovies, lake trout, white fish, herring, and albacore tuna provides at least one gram of omega-3 fatty acids. Farm-raised as opposed to wild-caught salmon can have significant levels of PCBs (cancer-causing environmental chemicals) and therefore should be eaten in moderation. Alpha-linolenic acid (ALA), another type of omega-3 fat found in plant foods such as flaxseed, hemp seeds, seaweed, walnuts, and soy bean and canola oil, can be converted in small amounts to EPA and DHA as a way to increase the total amount of healthy omega-3s in the diet.

Supplementation with fish oil can be a problem because it may contain environmental contaminants such as PCBs or mercury depending on the types of fish and fish parts used. Cod liver oil is not a good choice because it contains large amounts of vitamins A and D, which can be toxic when taken in large doses. Today there are fish oil preparations with very low levels of environmental contaminants. If you are lucky and have access to a Trader Joe's or Whole Foods market, both have very reasonably priced products that are filtered to remove PCBs and heavy metals. These products are tested by an independent laboratory for quality assurance. We recommend 500 to 1,000 mg daily to improve erectile function. The Trader Joe's product ("Trader Darwin" molecularly distilled omega-3 fatty acids) provides 300 mg of EPA and 200 mg of DHA per soft gel capsule. Because it is not known what exact balance is best for healthy erections, you should look for a product with similar characteristics or order it through www.Erectile-Function.com. Trader Joe's now sells a 600-mg omega-3 capsule with the fishy odor removed, for a minimally increased cost.

The American Heart Association recommends the following as a guide for omega-3 fatty acid intake:

(1) Individuals without documented coronary heart disease (CHD) should consume a variety of fatty fish at least two times each week and foods that are rich in alpha-linolenic acid such as flaxseed, canola oil, and walnuts.

(2) Individuals with documented CHD should consume about one gram of EPA and DHA per day (preferably from fatty fish) or consult their physician to consider EPA and DHA (fish oil) supplementation.

(3) Individuals who need to lower triglycerides should take two to four grams of EPA and DHA supplementation per day with their physician's supervision.

Note: Individuals taking more than three grams of EPA and DHA supplements should do so only under the supervision of a physician due to possibility of excessive thinning of the blood, which could result abnormal bleeding. Smaller doses do not appear to alter blood clotting significantly however, and do not add to the blood thinning effects of low-dose aspirin.

> "After a few weeks on the omeg-3s I knew something was very different. One morning I got up to shave and I just couldn't stand it. I hopped back into bed for a "quickie" that turned out to be not so quick. Boy, did we have to rush to get me out of the door in time to not be late for work! That has never happened before in many years of marriage. It was a *very* good feeling." Anonymous

Folic Acid:

Folic acid is an important nutrient that enhances the production of NO, so it appears to be very important for erectile health. High levels are found in enriched cereal, lentils, pinto beans, asparagus, spinach, and avocado. Strawberries, cantaloupes, and melons are also good sources. For individuals not used to eating these foods, it is best to take 400 micrograms (0.4 mg, the recommended daily intake) as a supplement. Folic acid, which is available in most drug stores, also has benefits for preventing high blood pressure and for reducing heart attacks. However, there has been recent concern that excessive amounts might increase the risk of colon cancer, so higher amounts are not recommended.

Antioxidants:

Antioxidants help to protect the body from the harmful effects of free oxygen radicals (highly reactive compounds formed when the body burns calories). They also keep certain chemical reactions in the body going in the right direction. For example, the reaction that produces NO can either produce NO or, when not enough antioxidants are present, the reaction produces a substance called a superoxide radical instead of NO (see diagram below). In a study of men with ED, the amount of effective glutathione (an important intracellular antioxidant) was significantly decreased. This means that lower levels of some antioxidants are present in men with ED. Antioxidants also protect our DNA (the cell's genetic material) from becoming fragmented and therefore protect against the development of cancer.

The table below lists many natural sources of antioxidants and their relative amounts. It also allows you to assess your intake of these important compounds. A newly recognized potent antioxidant-containing fruit, pomegranate, has been recently shown by Dr. Ignarro to increase NO production by blood vessels, making it an important nutrient for erectile health.

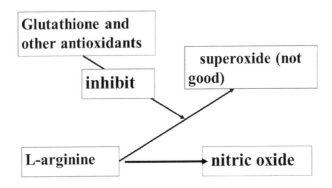

Adequate levels of antioxidants within the cell will maintain production of NO by preventing the formation of harmful superoxide. Certain antioxidants also protect NO from being destroyed by superoxide. Dr. Ignarro has shown, for example, that pomegranate juice is an extremely potent inactivator of the harmful superoxide.

Antioxidant Sources: (H = high, M = medium, L = low levels)

Pomegranate juice (4 oz.) H
Dark chocolate (1 oz.) H
Red wine (4 oz.) H
Blueberries (processed or fresh, 1 cup) H
Green or black tea (one cup) H
Blackberries (1 cup) H
Concord grape juice (regular dark purple) (1cup) H
White wine (4 oz.) M
Small red beans (dried, half cup) M
Red kidney beans (dried, half cup) M
Pinto beans (half cup) M
Cranberries (1 cup) M
Artichokes (cooked 1 cup) M
Prunes (half cup) M
Raspberries (1 cup) M

Strawberries (1 cup) M
Red delicious apple (1) M
Granny Smith apple (1) M
Pecans (1 oz.) M
Sweet cherries (1 cup) M
Black plums (1) M
Dark cherries M
Grapefruit juice (1 cup) M
Tomato juice (1 cup) M
Orange juice (1 cup) M
Vitamin C (500 mg) M
Vitamin E (200 IU) M
Mushrooms (1 cup) L
Red-skinned or russet potatoes (cooked, 1) L
Black beans (dried) half cup L
Plums (1) L
Gala apple (1) L
Apple juice (1 cup) L

A simpler way to ensure a good level of antioxidants is to regularly consume foods that contain high levels of these nutrients. Chocolate, red wine, blueberries, blackberries, tea (particularly green tea), pomegranate juice, and Concord grape juice have high levels. Any food that is colorful, such as fruits and vegetables, is also likely to be a good source of antioxidants. To obtain the most benefit, it is important to eat the skins of these colorful foods. Be careful that you don't also consume a lot of extra sugar, because good antioxidant sources are sometimes bitter tasting and some products have added sugar for better taste. Trader Joe's carries good tasting low sugar dark chocolates. They also have a Concord grape juice that has healthier artificial sweeteners. It is also best to add NutraSweet or Splenda rather than sugar when you need to sweeten your tea.

"After increasing my intake of folic acid, omega-3s, and antioxidants, we were on a vacation and after having had a great meal of white fish the previous evening we just stayed in bed the next day like honeymooners. We've occasionally made love two or three times in a day when on vacation, but five times? That day was better than we had ever experienced, even on our real honeymoon many, many years ago." Anonymous

Calcium:

Intracellular calcium is an important factor in the production of NO. Although it is not known whether the proper level of calcium intake will influence NO production, there are other reasons for getting enough of this important mineral. The main reason for consuming enough calcium throughout life is to optimize the levels of calcium in bone to add strength. Both men and women can lose significant bone density with increasing age. Osteoporosis (bones weakened by not enough calcium) occurs more commonly in women but can also occur in men. This may result in back and other deformities and even dangerous fractures.

There have been many studies that examine the possible benefit of calcium for lowering blood pressure and there appears to be some benefit.

A recent study that examined calcium intake in obese individuals who were on a 300 to 400 mg calcium/weight loss diet had some interesting findings. Some of the obese subjects in the study received an additional 800 mg of calcium as a supplement in tablet form and others received enough dairy products in their diet to increase calcium intake to 1,200 mg. Greater losses of weight, particularly abdominal fat, occurred when subjects got their extra calcium from the diet compared to calcium supplementation in tablet form. Calcium and milk proteins in the diet appear to reduce fat accumulation in fat cells.

Below is a list indicating the main dietary sources of calcium so that you can see how much you are getting in your diet.

Calcium Sources:

Evaporated milk, canned (fat-free) (4 oz. or ½ cup) 370 mg
Yogurt (plain, fruit, low-fat, fat-free) (1 cup) 300-400 mg
Swiss, gruyere cheese (1 oz.) 70 mg
Dry milk powder (fat-free) (1 tbsp.) 52 mg
Milk or buttermilk (8 oz. or 1 cup) 280-300 mg
Burrito, tostada, or enchilada with cheese (1 medium) 150-200 mg
Cheddar or mozzarella cheese (1 oz.) 200 mg
Cheeseburger (1) 200 mg
Custard (½ cup) 150 mg
Lasagna, frozen (1 cup) 200 mg
Ricotta cheese (low-fat, part-skim, whole (¼ cup) 150 mg
Salmon, canned with bones (3 oz.) 180-205 mg
Soybeans, roasted (1 cup) 200 mg
Beans (baked, small white, pinto, great northern) (1 cup) 150 mg
American cheese (1 oz.) 150 mg
Greens, cooked (turnip, mustard, dandelion, beet) (1 cup) 90-120 mg
Parmesan cheese, fresh, shredded (2 tbsp.) 140 mg
Pudding, flan (½ cup) 150 mg
Almonds (1 oz., 24 whole) 70 mg
Beans (chick peas, lima) (1 cup) 100 mg
Cottage cheese (½ cup) 75 mg
Cream cheese (fat-free) (2 tbsp.) 25 mg

Flour tortilla (1 medium, 10-in.) 100 mg
Greens, cooked (chard, kale) (1 cup) 100 mg
Ice cream, frozen yogurt (½ cup) 85-120 mg
Macaroni and cheese, from box (1 cup) 100-150 mg
Pizza, cheese (1 slice, ⅛ of 12 in.) 100-120 mg
Waffle or pancake (4-6 in.) 100 mg
Broccoli, cooked (½ cup) 70 mg
Corn tortilla (1 medium, 6 in.) 50 mg
Orange (1 medium, 3 in.) 50 mg
Sour cream (fat-free) (2 tbsp.) 50 mg

As you can see, there are many good dietary sources of calcium. After considering whether you are consuming enough of these calcium-containing foods to meet your total daily need of about 1,000 to 1,200 mg., a simple guideline is to add more calcium if needed to meet the total by taking in two or three servings of dairy every day, such as milk, yogurt, cheese, or ice cream. You can ensure better bone health (and perhaps a better love life and a slightly lower blood pressure) by taking a supplement if there is any doubt that you are meeting your total daily need from diet alone. It is not a good idea to double up on multi-vitamins with calcium to get more calcium. If you do this you could be getting too much vitamin A (the retinol form) or too much iron, both of which can be toxic. For men, it is best to take 1,200 mg or less of calcium daily, because higher amounts (1,500 mg or more) may increase your risk for prostate cancer, and in a recent study in women taking a calcium supplements who were already consuming at least 800 mg the supplements were associated with a higher risk of heart attack.

Good nutrition is about a lot more than good erections. Improving overall health leads to a longer life and more opportunities to take advantage of your firmer erections. Although the expanded book, available for download online, has more information about good nutrition, we would like to emphasize here the importance of fiber and healthy types of fat in your diet.

Fiber:

Although something that is not completely digested sounds like it ought to be bad for you, fiber (the indigestible component of food) is good for you and important for reducing colon and breast cancer and heart disease. It also helps to prevent diverticulosis (false passages in the intestines) and constipation. Foods rich in fiber include veggies, fruits, and whole grains (found in whole wheat bread and some cereals, such as oatmeal, oat bran, muesli, Total, shredded wheat, bran flakes, and brown rice and legumes). Brown basmati rice and "quick-cooking" brown rice are now available.

We recommend that you also try some other whole grains such quinoa, whole wheat couscous (pronounced koos koos), and whole grain bulgur instead of white rice. One cup of cooked whole grain bulgur has 150 calories, whereas 1 cup of cooked white rice provides 205 calories. The whole grain bulgur also has the added benefits of fiber (approximately 8 grams in 1 cup), vitamins, minerals, antioxidants, and other good things such as phytochemicals. Soluble fiber (fiber that goes into solution) has further benefits in binding harmful fatty acids and prolonging emptying time from the stomach so that sugar and carbohydrates are absorbed at a healthier rate. Soluble fiber reduces LDL cholesterol (the bad kind) and also small particles of lipoproteins (fatty substances) that can clog blood vessels. Good sources of soluble fiber are oats and oat bran, beans, peas, broccoli, brussel sprouts, barley, flax seed, carrots, apples, oranges, and psyllium as in Bran Buds cereal. Other whole grain products include pasta made from whole wheat, spelt, or kamut. Fiber also helps you fill up and therefore feel more satisfied with fewer calories. Our website has information on how you can include some whole grains in your favorite recipes.

Fat

Although all fats provide nine calories per gram, more than the four calories per gram that proteins and carbohydrates provide, they can be differentiated on the basis of healthy and not so healthy. There are two general categories of fat—saturated and unsaturated. The unhealthiest are saturated fats and trans fats (trans fats occur artificially when oils are processed to give them a longer shelf life and to make them more solid). Both of these types of fat are known to increase heart disease and a number of cancers. Saturated fats are typically found in animal fat, but some are from plant sources (tropical oils such as coconut, palm, and palm kernel). Unfortunately, they are difficult to avoid because they are present in most processed foods. The recommended amount of saturated fat is 10 percent or less of total calories. The healthiest fats are from the unsaturated category (monounsaturated fats and polyunsaturated fats) and are found primarily in plant sources (canola oil, olive oil, other vegetable oils, avocados, nuts). Among the unsaturated fats, monounsaturated and omega-3 fatty acids are considered to be the most "heart" and erection healthy. Good sources of monounsaturated fats include canola and olive oils.

Trans fats deserve special mention because of their strong link to heart disease. The food industry has used them extensively and preferentially because they cause oils to be more solid and manageable in food preparation and because foods made with trans fats do not spoil as easily. Trans fats have a much greater negative impact than saturated fat on the LDL/HDL cholesterol ratio (which pre-dicts the risk of heart disease). It has been estimated that trans fats are responsible for between 30,000 and 100,000 premature deaths from heart disease each year in the U.S. Several European countries have banned their use and some cities in the U.S. are now considering similar regula-tion. An increase of 2 percent of total calories from trans fat has been linked to a 40 percent increase of type 2 diabetes!

In addition to being present in most processed foods, they are present in most fried foods, because food provid-ers usually use trans fat-laden vegetable oils for deep frying. Don't be fooled by being told a particular restaurant uses vegetable oil rather than lard, because the trans fat and sat-urated fat content of some vegetable oils may be just as high as the level of saturated fat in lard. One well-known national food chain has admitted that one-third of the fat calories in their French fries are from trans fat. Getting voluntary cooperation of industry to reduce trans fat can be very dif-ficult. McDonald's announced that they would reduce trans fat in their cooking oil by 48 percent by February of 2003. However, on November 30, 2004, their website explained postponement of the change with the following statement: "While speedy implementation (of our trans fat reduction) is an admirable goal, we are most focused on the satisfac-tion of our customers and the quality of our products."

As of November 2004, Canada joined many European countries in efforts to reduce trans fat to the lowest possi-ble level. Hopefully these policies will spread to the U.S. by example, by consumer demand, or because it will be less expensive to manufacture food products one healthier way. At least now it is required in the U.S. for nutritional labels to include the amount of trans fat so that the con-sumer can be aware. You should know, however, that man-ufacturers and food producers do not have to list amounts that are less than half a gram per portion. Depending on the meal size (often a "portion" is not enough for a full meal), you still may be consuming too much. Look at the ingredient list, and if hydrogenated vegetable oil is present, avoid that product.

Cholesterol is a component of many foods in our diet. Our body also makes cholesterol (primarily in the liver). The body uses cholesterol to make several important hormones. On the negative side, excess cholesterol can be a major contributor to atherosclerosis (clogging of blood vessels), which can cause heart attacks and strokes. A reasonable amount of cholesterol in the diet (less than 300 mg per day is recommended by the American Heart Association) will not disturb your body's cholesterol level significantly. Dietary cholesterol is found only in animal products (dairy, meat, and eggs). You can reduce the amounts you consume by choosing low-fat or nonfat dairy products. Selecting lean cuts of meat and egg whites or an egg substitute such as "Eggbeaters" can also be very helpful. Although shrimp has relatively little fat, the amount of cholesterol is high. Lobster and crab have moderate amounts of cholesterol. However, all seafood, including shrimp, is a good choice of protein because of the low level of saturated fat. In fact, a study of normal individuals on a high shrimp diet (10 oz. per day) showed no increase in total cholesterol and favorable changes of the total cholesterol/HDL and LDL/HDL ratios and lower triglyceride levels. Check with your physician about whether you need to limit foods containing a lot of cholesterol based on measurements of your body's blood lipid (fat) levels.

Some Scientific Evidence Supporting this Chapter

1) What Color is Your Diet: The 7 Colors of Health, by David Heber, M.D., PhD, available on Amazon.com

2) Zemel MB, et al.: Calcium and dairy acceleration of weight and fat loss during energy restriction in obese adults. Obes Res 2004; 12: 582

3) www.americanheart.org/presenter. jhtml?identifier=3013797

4) Soluble fiber: www.healthandage.com/Home/ gid2=1080

5) Litin L, Sacks F Trans-fatty-acid content of common foods. N Engl J Med 1993; 329:1969.

I hadn't heard from pilot Ted for a while and, being curious whether it had helped to add the vitamin C, I thought I would see how he was doing. Based on further research, I also suggested adding 100 mg of Pycnogenol and 2 gm each of L-arginine and L-citrulline (see Chapter 7). He responded with the following e-mail:

It is good to hear from you. Hope all is well in the Meldrum compound. I am sorry to report that I am still manually hand propping my aircraft. I have a hot rod machine to fly with no hangar to put it in. You may use me for your book (anonymous, of course). I will also try out your recommendation. It sure feels good when the engine warms up and wakes me up in the morning ready for some action. You will be the first I contact when I get out of this slump I'm in.

"Ted"

Chapter Seven

Improving Your Erectile Health Naturally and Safely

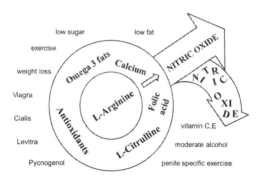

Now that you understand what makes your penis work, how can you get yours to be as solid as the science behind NO and erectile health?

First, realize that ED may be a symptom of an unhealthy vascular system or a more serious disease. Have an evaluation by your primary care physician or internist and a urologist. They will evaluate your heart and blood pressure and order tests to rule out diabetes and to measure your blood lipids. If you are overweight, they will suggest weight loss. If you smoke, they can suggest nicotine skin patches and possibly a medication called Zyban to help you quit. If you are inactive, they can check your health status before you embark on an exercise program. Weight loss will reverse most of the effects of excess weight on erectile health. It will lower your blood sugar levels and make your body more responsive to insulin. These beneficial effects will improve the NO production by your blood vessels. A lower-fat diet will result in lower circulating fatty acids and more NO synthesis as well. A urologist can examine your prostate and genitals and may measure your level of testosterone to detect any abnormalities indicating specific treatments.

Start with the factors that are natural, have proven effects on NO production, and also have definite cardiovascular benefits. Folic acid and omega-3 fats will reduce your chance of cardiovascular disease in the future while also improving your love life. Take about 1,000 mg of calcium per day, which will also help you lose weight, may lower your blood pressure slightly, and will help to ensure strong, healthy bones as you age. Increase your intake of natural antioxidants, which will also reduce heart disease and cancer. Give all of these things (including weight loss, lower dietary fat and sugar, and more activity) a few weeks to work and you may find that these changes are all that are necessary to solve your problem. If you are not fond of the various natural antioxidants described in this book, you can take 500 mg of vitamin C and 200 units of vitamin E daily.

If you need more help or if you just want to "push the envelope" on sexual performance, add a stronger antioxidant and a combination of L-arginine and L-citrulline: Pycnogenol, an effective antioxidant scavenger of superoxide, has been shown to increase NO production, and was very effective in a study of men with ED. Take 50 to 120 mg per day. The optimum doses of L-arginine and L-citrul-line have not been worked out. Two to three grams of each per day are reasonable doses (a total of five grams is in Dr. Ignarro's "Nite-Works" supplement for optimal blood vessel NO production and cardiovascular health).

> "We've all heard the expression "getting a hard on," but how hard is hard? Even if you got an experienced second opinion, she probably wouldn't deflate you by saying she's had a lot better. But you do know when you experience it. After trying all of the above, it's been much harder than I've ever experienced throughout my life. Many times it's been so hard that it is impossible to imagine it being any harder. Now I really do know how hard, hard is!" Anonymous

Is there any downside to all of this? No treatment that changes behavior can be all good. Some men's partners might not be receptive to their renewed interest and capability, and it certainly can disturb one's sleep when you awaken in the middle of the night with something that demands attention or will otherwise keep you awake. However, we feel that the increased capability for a couple to have a fully satisfying sex life will help enormously in keeping their relationship strong. If only one divorce can be prevented, with all of its consequences spinning out to involve children, friends, and loved ones, this book will have been worthwhile, and we think that many, many relationships will be cemented by maintaining or restoring what a couple has enjoyed together in the past.

If all of these factors do not yield a fully satisfactory result, pay particular attention to stress, personal habits, and your relationship with your partner. Stress and fatigue can be hard to change, but you may be able to dramatically improve your love life and your general health by taking on fewer tasks, modifying the situation at work or at home to make it less stressful, and getting more sleep. It's hard to have a fulfilling love life if you are not getting along with your partner. You may wish to see a marriage or family counselor. A sex therapist can also be helpful. Remember that lovemaking is not just a mechanical exercise. Sexual arousal is crucial to the physical changes and increased blood flow necessary for good sex. Both partners have to appreciate the importance of foreplay, and as a man ages, this becomes as important for him as it has always been for the female partner. A romantic evening or a different environment such as a weekend away alone can set the stage for turning a sexual problem around.

If all else fails, Viagra-like drugs will be much more likely to work if you have improved the ability of your blood vessel linings to make enough NO. Think of a simple analogy of a hose connected to a water outlet and terminating in a device to regulate outflow. You can markedly cut down on outflow (PDE5 inhibitors like Viagra reduce the breakdown of cyclic GMP), but if very little water is coming into the hose, it may remain limp. By opening the tap (turning on NO production), much more NO and cyclic GMP will be produced and more will accumulate, just as more flow of water will distend the hose and make it more rigid. Clearly working at this problem from both ends will be much more effective than either alone. Simply trying to shore up cyclic GMP with drugs when there just isn't enough NO being produced to stimulate cyclic GMP levels is much less likely to work or to work well enough for men to want to use a drug very often (particularly considering its expense).

The really incredible part of all of this is that every man has an indicator of his cardiovascular health right

there between his legs! Keeping your blood vessels elastic, relaxed, and capable of providing the blood flow that various parts of the body need will improve your general health and help to prevent heart attacks, strokes, and senility. Recent animal studies suggest that you may even be able to heal the effects of past poor nutrition and lifestyle by maximizing NO production If you follow all of the recommendations in Dr. Louis Ignarro's book entitled *No More Heart Disease*—exercise, weight control, a low-fat and low-sugar diet, good nutrition, supplements as needed—and particularly if you are then experiencing firm erections, you can be confident you are doing everything you can to keep your heart and blood vessels healthy. Of course you need to treat any remaining high blood pressure or abnormal blood lipids that may have a genetic or other known cause. Unfortunately, some people will have ignored their health for so long that even heart surgery may be required. But the vast majority of people can maintain their cardiovascular health without any of the inconvenience, cost, complications and side effects of drugs or surgery. Your health is truly in your hand!

Every story should have a happy ending, so I contacted Ted since I hadn't heard from him in a while. He sent this e-mail:

Dr. Meldrum,

I am so glad to hear from you. I was just about to contact you for an update. I now have a girlfriend!

My girlfriend has commented that our time together keeps getting better and better every time we make love. There was one time where she wanted me to make love to her again shortly after we just finished our last session. I was a little nervous; it has been a long time since I have given in multiple times. I was greatly surprised to find myself rising up for the occasion and she was pleasantly satisfied with my performance. I am not used to receiving compliments for my performances in bed. This is new for me.

My girlfriend thanks you and so do I. You're recipe is the greatest in more ways than one.

Ted

Although not mentioned above, Ted no longer uses any prescription medications for ED!

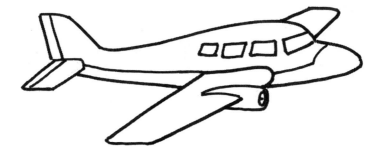

Chapter Eight

Here's Where the Trouble Starts

No man would doubt that the number one contributor to an erection is sexual arousal. Knowledge of the physiology only reinforces this fact. The nerves supplying the penile artery release NO, which causes a rapid relaxation of the smooth muscle in the wall of the penile artery and a marked increase of blood flow causing engorgement and erection. That is why, for a man, the mere thought of something erotic or a visually sexual stimulus can produce that "turned on" feeling. When that ability to respond declines due to age, obesity, inactivity, and a diet low in the nutrients that enhance NO production, a man feels, well, less than a man. At times it can feel kind of dead down there. And because a man's self-esteem is very much tied to his sexual potency, it's no wonder that the natural inclination is for him to look for ways to fix the problem.

Here is where the real trouble starts. The easiest fix is to seek stronger sexual stimuli. If it's a sexually stimulating video or magazine and nothing more, no problem, unless his partner takes offence and feels less desirable because he seems to need something more than her. Unfortunately those stronger stimuli may present themselves in the form of other women. Hence so many personal catastrophes that have ended in pain for loved ones, divorce, or even altered the course of nations. We are all familiar with prominent politicians and celebrities who have formed new and dangerous relationships, resulting in public humiliation of their wives and families. We all probably have friends who are doing the same without as much publicity. And some readers may be doing it themselves. Fixing the problem of decreased erectile function by applying the knowledge gained from this book and our website (erectile-function. com) can help to preserve an existing relationship that was once full of romance and love.

Presumably all these men and women really enjoyed their sexual relationship many years before when they were first married, and for years afterward. The key is to preserve or restore that same relationship and sexual enjoyment and not be lured by new sexual opportunities into personal disaster. Of course relationships and individual personalities are far more complex, but the premise of this book is that improved male sexual function can go a long way toward keeping relationships and families from being torn apart. The effect on happiness and self-esteem will have further spin-offs in one's work and other personal relationships, and a man's partner will feel more desired and will experience more sexual pleasure.

Viagra and similar drugs have revolutionized the field of erectile dysfunction and have helped many millions of couples. However, studies of these drugs have shown mainly a mechanical effect. These medications work by blocking the breakdown of cyclic GMP and have less impact on NO. By increasing NO through all of the recommendations in this book, sexual stimuli will produce those old familiar yearnings, making you feel younger as well as more potent. If further help is needed, you will be much more likely to respond to Viagra-like drugs. As if that isn't enough, you also will have a healthier heart and blood vessels, and you will decrease your risk of cancer.

People joke about a man following the organ between his legs instead of the one on top of his shoulders, but it is far from being a joke. You can follow it to personal disaster, as many men have, or you can use your head and follow a path that will strengthen the relationship most important to you and improve your health at the same time. Now that's a no-brainer!

Epilogue – Where Did We All Begin?

With an erection, of course. If not for this vital function, none of us would be here! Whether by grand design or evolution, the physiologic process through which an erection occurs had to be designed so that it would reliably occur under widely varied circumstances during early man's existence.

As all of the factors influencing NO became apparent, it seemed remarkable to us that they were all related to various sources of energy—omega-3s from fish; antioxidants, vitamin C and E and nitrate from fruits, vegetables, and nuts; calcium from dairy; L-arginine from various sources of protein; and from a variety of foods that stimulate insulin. Such a complex system with many redundant mechanisms makes sense. No matter how varied early man's diet was in different locales and with changing climates, some form of energy would likely have been available to stimulate NO enough for an erection to occur. Food was never plentiful enough for a man to become obese. Even meat sources were lean. And the only sugar would have been the low amounts present in fruit. It also makes sense that a fit and lean body would be connected to better NO production and therefore better erections. If early man was in good physical condition, which requires lots of exercise, he would have been more able to protect his pregnant mate and offspring from predators. On the other hand, if the supply of energy was extremely poor, procreation would have been better served by delaying pregnancy until circumstances improved, so the nutritional demands of pregnancy and breast feeding could be met.

It seemed abundantly clear to us that the complex biochemistry of NO production evolved for one purpose—reproduction! This entirely new theory was first put forth by us in a review published in December 2010 entitled "A multifaceted approach to maximize erectile function and vascular health" (PMID: 20522326). Many reading this theory for the first time will probably say "of course." As Lou Ignarro said in his foreword to this book, just as with the discovery of Velcro or Zip-Lock bags, one only has to examine our theory to believe it is true.

We all can benefit from this knowledge by realizing that these numerous ways to stimulate NO give us a remarkable capacity to improve both erectile function and vascular health. But how long can such a good thing last? We alluded in the first chapter to another process of discovery by an explorer named Dan Buettner. Dan has travelled with a team of scientists from the National Geographic Society to places in the world where unusual proportions of men and women not only live into their nineties or even over one hundred, but have remarkable health. After writing about "The Blue Zones" in a national best seller of that title, his team visited another such area off the coast of Greece, an island called Ikaria. In his book you will see that exercise, a lean body, and lots of vegetables and fruits were common to all these regions. And here's the kicker—in a survey of men living in Ikaria who were over age ninety, averaging ninety-five, 70 percent said they were still sexually active. So apparently it can last for a very long time!

With any new way of approaching an old problem, even one so extensively backed up by science as we have documented here and in our two published reviews, there will still be some "doubting Thomases." However, here we have an entirely unique situation. Virtually every sexually active adult is both interested in this subject and capable of their own experiment. It is always difficult for any man to know how good he is at this. Most of us have no real basis of comparison, and even if your partner seems to be really enjoying it, she could be pulling a "Meg Ryan" (if you haven't seen the diner scene in *When Harry Met Sally* where she noisily fakes an orgasm for a skeptical Billy Crystal, you must have been living on another planet!). What any man (or woman) will know, though, is whether he is better. For me and for my partner of over forty years, we are enjoying our sexual relationship now much more than when we were first together, and we are both over sixty-five. So to any "doubting Thomas" we would simply say "try it."

Authors' Notes

1) Exercise, exercise, exercise

It is difficult to overemphasize the importance of exercise. Lou Ignarro was first to show that increased blood flow stimulates production of NO in the endothelium of blood vessels (PMID: 1991651). The increased flow crinkles the surface membrane of those cells, which releases calcium that in turn stimulates NO production. The involvement of calcium is probably the reason that calcium supplements reduce blood pressure, particularly in individuals whose calcium intake is deficient (PMID: 16673011). Daily exercise is very important. While a single episode of exercise increases NO for about forty-eight hours, daily exercise causes a four-fold increase of NO that lasts for about a week (PMID: 16874149). Exercise also increases the activity of an important circulating antioxidant, para-oxinase-1 [PMID:12798217] that is decreased in men with ED.

Exercise also increases NO production in response to insulin. Insulin is a principal stimulator of NO. In one study, the production of NO in response to insulin increased by two-thirds following twelve weeks of exercise training (PMID: 16889802).

ED is associated with sedentary activity and with hours of television viewing as an indicator of inactivity (PMID: 17275456). Men who are sedentary are two to three times more likely to have ED (PMID: 12899583). Moderate exercise reduces ED by two-thirds, and a high level of exercise reduces ED by over 80 percent (PMID: 12180232).

2) Omega-3 fatty acids

A supplement of omega-3s may be the single most important stimulator of erectile function. The omega-3 fats even stimulate another factor that may be involved in penile engorgement, the vasodilating prostaglandins. This was not discussed in our review that concentrated on the role of NO, but as you learned in this book, prostaglandin E is used to aid erection as a suppository placed into the penile opening. Because it would be difficult to obtain 500 to 1,000 mg of omega-3s per day from the diet (except perhaps in Scandinavian countries), a fish oil supplement is generally used to provide these amounts. There is a prescription form that cardiologists might prefer because it is more standardized, but fish oil is most likely equally effective. Just one bit of caution, though. The omega-3 fats are themselves very sensitive to oxidation and therefore are best taken along with large amounts of antioxidants. They will be more effective, and some concern (without evidence) has been expressed that increased amounts of omega-3s could be harmful without being protected from oxidation by a good level of antioxidants.

3) Antioxidants

Antioxidants may be as important as the omega-3s, and as pointed out above, the two are best taken as a combined treatment. The strongest antioxidants are the polyphenols that are present in large amounts in pomegranate (PMID: 16626982), green tea PMID: (16872562), berries (PMID: 19298192), chocolate (PMID: 14654748), and red wine (PMID: 12575978). Antioxidants not only increase the production of NO, but also prevent its breakdown (PMID: 16626982). It does appear that men with ED are deficient in their intracellular antioxidant defenses. The level of reduced glutathione, one of the cells' most important natural antioxidants, is reduced in men with ED (PMID: 15910541). In another study, paraoxinase-1, possibly the most important circulating antioxidant, was markedly lower in a study of young men with ED (PMID: 17554394).

Green tea is of particular benefit because it also has been associated with a marked decrease of prostate cancer. Prostate cancer is relatively rare in China (eighteen times less common than in the U.S.) and in one study, intake of three cups of green tea per day was associated with over 70 percent reduction of this cancer (PMID: 14618627). Men particularly fear prostate cancer because the treatments can cause ED that may not respond to usual treatments. Be aware that the decaffeination process removes various beneficial chemicals in addition to removing the caffeine. In one study drinking tea was associated with a significant reduction of a second heart attack (PMID: 12034652), showing that even unhealthy blood vessels respond with increased NO production. In that study cardiovascular mortality was reduced by almost 50 percent, a highly significant difference compared to non-tea drinkers.

Everyone knows that blueberries have lots of antioxidants, but in one study blackberries had twice as much, and strawberries had an equal amount compared with blueberries (PMID: 16825686). Eating the whole fruit is best because the skins contain the largest amount of antioxidants.

Chocolate has very marked effects on NO production. In one study, even after five days of ingesting a large amount of cocoa that caused increased NO production, there was still a marked increase of NO ninety minutes after a "dose" (PMID: 14654748). Just as with tea, intake of chocolate was associated with reduced mortality following a first heart attack. Consumption of 50 grams twice or more per week was associated with a remarkable two-thirds reduction of mortality (PMID: 19711504). The chocolate was not specified to be dark chocolate, and usually chocolate also contains a substantial amount of sugar. A study of NO production with cocoa compared to cocoa plus sugar (the amount in a sugary soda) showed that sugar reversed about two-thirds of the benefit of the cocoa (PMID: 18614724).

These results on mortality are even more significant because the benefit of the cocoa was sufficient to have this dramatic effect even though it was partly offset by an adverse effect of sugar. Ideally a dark chocolate containing a high percentage of cocoa with a minimum of sugar should have the best effect on NO production. The best chocolate we have been able to find has 85 percent cocoa with only 6 grams of sugar in a 40 gram portion (Trader Joe's Dark Chocolate Lover's Chocolate Bar). A remarkably good taste is achieved by adding vanilla for extra flavor. As with most changes of food preferences, it's remarkable how a person's tastes change with any new form of nutrition, and I now enjoy this newest find more than less concentrated chocolate containing more sugar.

Red wine has high levels of polyphenols. Also, mild to moderate alcohol stimulates both vascular NO (PMID: 16043025) and the good fraction of cholesterol (HDL) and is associated with less ED (PMID: 17538641). Although we would not want to encourage anyone to start drinking alcohol, it is difficult to get so many benefits from something that can also give that much pleasure. Beer, on the other hand, contains less antioxidant, and the maltose is converted to more sugar than is present in a comparable amount of wine. It may be the stimulation of insulin that results in the typical abdominal fat deposition ("beer belly") of beer drinkers. It is clear from many cardiovascular and ED studies that central fat deposition is linked to both ED and cardiovascular disease.

Fruits and vegetables also contain antioxidants. Almost without exception, cooking of vegetables (and fruits such as tomato) increases the amount of antioxidant (PMID: 16825686). However, the amount of antioxidant is still far less than in berries. The decrease of certain vitamins with cooking of vegetables is generally not significant in someone ingesting the recommended number of vegetable servings. It has even recently been found that the nitrate in vegetables, previously thought to be bad for health, appears to increase NO (PMID: 20876122). Investigators found that nitrate ingestion by NO-deficient animals similar to the amount present in recommended portions of vegetables increased NO and also decreased abdominal fat, pre-diabetes, and blood pressure. In the book *The Blue Zones*, author Dan Buettner describes the factors common to unique areas around the world where people live longer and healthier lives. You guessed it—a high intake of vegetables was common to every one of those areas.

Two commercial antioxidants that have been shown to benefit erectile function in well-designed studies are pycnogenol and ginseng. Pycnogenol contains polyphenols similar to those in berries, and it is well-standardized and its antioxidant properties have been extensively investigated, whereas ginseng is available in so many different preparations that it is difficult to be sure regarding efficacy of a particular product. We therefore suggest pycnogenol, in a dose of 80 to 120 mg, for those who would rather take capsules than consume the foods we have recommended. It is less expensive than a comparable dose of antioxidant from berries.

What about vitamin C and vitamin E? They are antioxidants, but they're thirty to fifty times less potent than the various sources of polyphenols discussed above. If large amounts are taken (for example, 1,000 mg of vitamin C and 800 mg of vitamin E as in the study on smokers below) similar benefits might be expected, and they work together, each increasing the circulating levels of the other (PMID: 10967604). However, we recommend taking no more than 200 IU of vitamin E, because larger amounts have been associated with an increase of all-cause mortality (PMID: 15537682). Furthermore, vitamin E should be avoided entirely for anyone taking aspirin. Vitamin E markedly increases the anti-platelet effect of aspirin, which could cause a serious bleeding episode. In physicians who were taking 400 IU every other day, a significant increase of hemorrhagic stroke was observed (PMID: 18997197). Many older men, and particularly physicians, take low-dose aspirin. Larger doses of vitamin C are apparently innocuous but could cause heartburn. We would ask why take these weak antioxidants when much better ones are readily available, and can even be enjoyed? They are, however, inexpensive and are a good alternative for someone with a limited budget. Substituting green tea for other more costly beverages and taking 1,000 mg of vitamin C and 200 IU of vitamin E provides the best antioxidant "bang for the buck."

4) Folic acid

Folic acid, or folate, plays an important role in the production of NO. The recommended daily allowance (RDA) is 400 micrograms, and deficient intake is common. Folic acid has been identified as a factor that prevents hypertension (high blood pressure), and some studies have suggested that it helps to prevent colon cancer. It is reasonable to take a 400 microgram supplement—although there has been some recent concern that excessive folic acid could stimulate existing colon cancer. If your intake is already high, a supplement may not be necessary. Natural sources of folate are green leafy vegetables, nuts, beans, peas, and avocado. Folic acid is also added to cereals and bread.

5) Penile-specific exercise

In a study in Finland, men who had more frequent intercourse were half as likely to develop ED (PMID: 18538297). That makes sense because the increase of blood flow in the penis with erection is many times the increase of blood flow in systemic arteries with exercise. The shear stress known to markedly increase NO production in the lining of blood vessels with increased blood flow (discussed above) would be expected to be even more prominent in the penile vessels, although the duration of the increased blood flow is of course shorter. It would appear that the better the quality of the erection and the longer the erection lasts, the more effect it will have on future erectile performance.

Empirically that is what is observed. As function improves, it appears to further improve over time and can be sustained to a remarkable extent. Hugh Hefner, eighty-four, was engaged to be married to a woman sixty years his junior. In a survey of men over age ninety (averaging ninety-five) on the Greek island of Ikaria, where an unusual number of people live into their nineties or even to over one hundred, 70 percent said they were still sexually active. The inhabitants of Ikaria follow most of the things we recommend in this book, with exercise and eating cooked green vegetables being the most prominent examples.

The flip side of the "use it or lose it" dictum is that disuse would be expected to lead to progressively poorer function. In fact, "penile rehabilitation" is now well-supported as being critical to preserving erectile function following surgical treatment of prostate cancer, by using a vacuum device (PMID: 20410903) and/or PDE-5 inhibitors (PMID: 20156044). Likewise during any hiatus between relationships, exercising "George" every day or two may improve performance when sexual activity resumes. It may well be that nocturnal erections have played an important role during evolution when the daily life challenges of early man may not have left opportunities for sexual activity.

Above are the five most important factors aiding erectile performance, and it is difficult to say which is more important. The next five are less critical, only apply to certain men, and some may be more difficult to change.

6) Don't smoke

NO is a very unstable compound. It's made up of an atom of nitrogen connected to an atom of oxygen, but the bond between them allows it to be readily broken down. It can also be changed to other compounds that are bad for blood vessel health that break down NO and inhibit its production. It's remarkable that such an unstable system evolved to maintain a function upon which the very survival of humanity depends. The production of NO is promoted by anti-oxidants and inhibited by oxidation products called free oxygen radicals.

Smoking exposes the blood vessels to substances that prevent the normal production of NO through oxidative stress and formation of the very toxic compounds superoxide and peroxinitrite. The marked decrease of NO is what causes ED and increases cardiovascular disease in smokers (even second-hand smoke has been linked to ED) (PMID: 10731462). One would therefore predict that antioxidants might prevent these problems in smokers, and in fact from one remarkable study (PMID: 19363134), that appears to be the case. In this excellent study that should have been in a top medical journal, smoking was found to markedly suppress NO production (NO is assessed in a subject by measuring the reactive blood flow in the forearm following constriction then release of the blood supply; this "flow-mediated dilation" (FMD) is due to NO and is a common research measurement in this field). Even more importantly, high doses of vitamin C (1,000 mg) and vitamin E (800 IU) completely restored NO production. Vitamins C and E are weak antioxidants, and we do not recommend taking more than 200 IU of vitamin E, but this study established that antioxidants can help to reverse the ED and heart disease due to smoking. Of course, the longer someone has smoked, the more irreversible changes may be present in their blood vessels.

7) Don't drink excessive alcohol

Mild to moderate alcohol stimulates, but excessive alcohol suppresses NO production by the blood vessel lining (PMID: 16043025). In the penis, excessive alcohol actually causes those NO-producing lining cells to undergo structural changes, although the release of NO from the penile nerves remains unchanged (PMID: 19066420). This explains why an inebriated person may still be able to perform as long as he has enough sexual arousal to stimulate NO release by the nerves supplying the penile blood vessels.

8) Lose extra weight, particularly if the weight is concentrated in the abdomen

Abdominal fat causes resistance to the body's insulin, and insulin is a major stimulator of NO. Obesity and the waist/hip ratio (a good index of abdominal obesity) are strongly correlated with ED (PMID: 15505991), while weight loss and decreased abdominal fat improve erectile function. Katherine Esposito, a co-author of our review, her mentor Dario Giugliano, and their team of researchers in Naples, Italy, have done the best work on the metabolic causes of ED. In their classic paper in the prestigious *Journal of the American Medical Association*, they reported on a large group of obese men with ED who had significantly improved erectile function with weight loss and increased activity (PMID: 15213209).

In a study of obese men undergoing a program of diet and increased activity, reported in the equally prestigious journal *Circulation*, Roberts and co-workers showed that as their subjects' sensitivity to insulin increased, NO production also went up (PMID: 12427646). A low-carbohydrate diet (PMID: 20679559), together with exercise (PMID: 17301622), should be the most effective approach for improving erectile function. Each is effective in decreasing blood pressure, which may be the most obvious index that an obese person can monitor, besides erectile function, to gauge improvement of his vascular health. An automated blood pressure cuff can be purchased in any pharmacy.

9) L-arginine or L-citrulline

If you search online for erectile dysfunction you will find lots of sites selling L-arginine, usually at ineffective doses. L-arginine is the direct precursor of NO, but it's extensively metabolized in the bowel and liver. The average amount present in a normal diet is about 5 grams. Studies on ED have shown no benefit at a dose of 1.5 grams, which makes sense because that dose would be small relative to the amount in a normal diet. To achieve any detectable effect requires a dose of 5 grams, which would double the amount that is normally ingested per day. L-citrulline requires about half as much to achieve the same circulating level of L-arginine. Therefore a dose of 2 to 3 grams of L-citrulline would be expected to have a positive effect. However, in one study of men who were admitted with a heart attack, 9 grams of L-arginine per day *appeared* to increase mortality (a study may be stopped when it is not certain that the occurrence of a complication is statistically significant because of the seriousness of the event, as was the case here). NO is involved in inflammation and therefore we would suggest not taking either of these supplements during any severe illness.

10) Decrease the amount of sugar and fat in your diet

Sugar decreases NO. The only difference between a juvenile diabetic and a normal individual is that they have higher circulating glucose levels. Juvenile diabetics develop severe early vascular disease unless their glucose levels are very carefully controlled. The amount of sugar ingested by people today is huge compared to fifty or one hundred years ago when sugar was a rare and expensive commodity. Today sugar is so inexpensive that it is many times more profitable for the food industry to add sugar for flavor compared to fat. If you examine nutrition labels carefully you will see high fructose corn syrup in a very wide range of food products, such that an average person could be considered a little bit diabetic. Some individuals take in so much sugar and simple carbohydrates that are rapidly converted to sugar that they will have premature vascular disease similar to an average juvenile diabetic.

Tragically, sugar has been found to be more addictive even than cocaine, so breaking the sugar habit can be difficult. We would recommend avoiding full sugar sodas and to eat whole fruit and avoid fruit juices. If you do partake in desserts, take one to three bites and stop. Pick food products with little or no sugar added, and avoid high-carb snacks. Any sugar that you do eat should be combined with fat and protein so it is slowly absorbed.

Fat also decreases NO production by blood vessels, and the average diet in the U.S. contains too much fat. Maintaining a low-fat diet has been found to be a characteristic of individuals who have been successful in losing weight and maintaining the loss. An easy way to reduce fat intake is to avoid all fried foods and fatty beef.

What about testosterone?

If all of the above recommendations fail to satisfactorily improve erectile function, you should have your physician measure your testosterone level. Testosterone stimulates NO, and NO falls as the circulating level of testosterone decreases. Even if the level is in the low normal range, testosterone treatment may be helpful. Studies have clearly shown in those instances that the response to the Viagra-like drugs can be restored. Testosterone is most often administered by a cream or a skin patch and should be monitored closely by a physician. Testosterone treatment can also decrease abdominal fat and increase the sensitivity of your body to insulin. The reason we suggest first maximizing NO is that in one study testosterone levels increased when a combination of eighty mg of the antioxidant pycnogenol and three grams of L-arginine were taken daily for one month (PMID: 17703218). By following our recommendations to maximize NO, increased blood flow to the testicles may normalize testosterone production.

Viagra-like drugs

We haven't discussed PDE-5 inhibitors like Viagra, Cialis, and Levitra because the ideal approach is to first do all of the above. Then if a PDE-5 is required, your response will be better and you will need lower doses.

I had begun this journey through the world's medical literature with the very strong notion that these drugs would just cover up the underlying poor vascular function rather than treating the underlying problem. However, most drugs have more than one effect on the body, and it turns out that these drugs improve the antioxidant status of the blood and tissues. A study done at peak blood levels after a 20 mg dose of Cialis showed that total serum antioxidants rose 45 percent, total serum oxidant status fell 33 percent, and serum paraoxinase-1 rose 50 percent (if you recall, PON-1 is one of the most important circulating natural antioxidants) and it is lower in men with ED.

Men with ED have decreased circulating and intracellular antioxidants, and antioxidants are essential for the production of NO and to protect it from being broken down. In a study done four weeks after taking a 20-mg dose of Cialis every other day, men with cardiovascular risk factors had marked increases of NO, and the levels were still elevated two weeks after stopping the drug. If you recall, we had indicated that these drugs act by blocking the breakdown of a cellular messenger called cyclic GMP. From animal studies it appears that cyclic GMP improves antioxidant status. It had even been shown that blood pressure was significantly reduced by taking 50 mg of Viagra three times daily. These drugs do have very favorable effects on blood vessel health and therefore we would encourage men to use them if they do not have a fully satisfactory response to methods one through ten above or by correcting a low testosterone level.

CAUTION: Very occasionally these drugs can cause a prolonged, painful erection requiring a trip to the emergency room for an injection into the penis to allow the erection to resolve. If you have increased the NO production by your blood vessels by following our recommendations this may be more likely to occur with usual doses of these drugs. Start at one-fourth of the usual dose and gradually increase once you are sure you are not over responding.

1. http://www.nlm.nih.gov/pubs/factsheets/loansome_doc.html
2. https://docline.gov/loansome/registerbegin.cfm?
3. Meldrum DR, Gambone JC, Morris MA, Meldrum, DAN, Esposito K, Ignarro, LJ. The link between erectile and vascular health: The canary in the coal mine. Amer J Cardiol 2011; e-pub ahead of print, 28 May 2011 [PMID:21624550]

Made in the USA
Lexington, KY
13 October 2012